Legal Handbook
for Pharmacy Technicians

Diane L. Darvey, Pharm.D., JD
Alexandria, VA

Editorial Content Advisor
W. Renee' Acosta, R.Ph., M.S.
Clinical Assistant Professor
Pharmacy Practice Division
College of Pharmacy
The University of Texas at Austin

American Society of Health-System Pharmacists
Bethesda, MD

Any correspondence regarding this publication should be sent to the publisher, American Society of Health-System Pharmacists, 7272 Wisconsin Avenue, Bethesda, MD 20814, attention: Special Publishing.

The information presented herein reflects the opinions of the contributors and advisors. It should not be interpreted as an official policy of ASHP or as an endorsement of any product. The information contained in this publication is to be used as guidance.

Because of ongoing changes in laws and regulations, the information and its applications contained in this text are constantly evolving and are subject to the professional judgment and interpretation of states and the circumstances of pharmacy practice. The editors, contributors, and ASHP have made reasonable efforts to ensure the accuracy and appropriateness of the information presented in this document. However, any user of this information is advised that the editors, contributors, advisors, and ASHP are not responsible for the continued currency of the information, for any errors or omissions, and/or for any consequences arising from the use of the information in the document in any and all practice settings. Any reader of this document is cautioned that ASHP makes no representation, guarantee, or warranty, express or implied, as to the accuracy and appropriateness of the information contained in this document and will bear no responsibility or liability for the results or consequences of its use.

Director, Special Publishing: Jack Bruggeman
Acquisitions Editor: Hal Pollard
Senior Editorial Project Manager: Dana Battaglia
Project Editor: Johnna Hershey
Cover Design: Jim DeVall
Page Design and Composition: Carol Barrer

Library of Congress Cataloging-in-Publication Data

Darvey, Diane L.
    Legal handbook for pharmacy technicians / Diane L. Darvey.
        p. cm.
    ISBN 978-1-58528-159-6
    1. Pharmacy--Law and legislation--United States. 2. Drugs--Law and legislation--United States. 3. Pharmacy technicians--Legal status, laws, etc.--United States. 4. Pharmacy technicians--United States--Handbooks, manuals, etc. 5. Pharmacists--Legal status, laws, etc.--United States. 6. Privacy, Right of--United States. I. Title.

    KF2915.P4D357 2008
    344.7304'16--dc22

                                                    2008005251

ISBN: 978-1-58528-159-6

Dedication

To my friends and colleagues:

"Education is the best provision for old age."
—Aristotle

Preface

The practice of pharmacy is growing steadily more complex. Medications have become increasingly essential to treating disease, and each year brings the introduction of ever more sophisticated drugs. Pharmacists have an essential role in medication use through counseling patients on proper medication use; advising physicians, nurses, and other health care providers on medication therapy management; and working collaboratively with physicians. It is no surprise that pharmacy is one of the most highly regulated health professions.

As pharmacists take on expanded roles in the health care system, the importance of pharmacy technicians is highlighted too. They have a key role in supporting pharmacists. Today, technicians do many of the tasks that only a few years ago were performed by the pharmacist.

Like the pharmacy profession itself, the laws and regulations of pharmacy are complex and changing. Each state has its own set of pharmacy laws and regulations. The sheer magnitude of all these laws and regulations makes it impossible to specifically address all of them. In this book, I have taken the approach of providing examples of state laws and regulations that illustrate those found in most states. This approach should provide a foundation for pharmacy technicians, or persons studying to become technicians, to understand how their particular state regulates pharmacy and pharmacy technicians. In the pages that follow, you will read about the laws and regulations applicable to pharmacy technicians such as whether pharmacy technicians must be registered as well as the qualifications to become a pharmacy technician.

For the pharmacy technician, understanding the laws and regulations of pharmacy is an essential part of doing your job and doing it well. The fact that pharmacy is so highly regulated is a clear sign of the importance of your job and the importance of the pharmacy profession to the health and well being of patients.

Diane Darvey
December 2007

Disclaimer

This publication has been prepared by the author for general informational purposes only and is not intended to contain all laws and regulations that relate or may relate to the practice of pharmacy, including but not limited to pharmacy technicians. This publication and the materials therein are not provided in the course of an attorney–client relationship and are not intended to provide legal or other advice. Such advice should only be rendered in reference to the particular facts and circumstances appropriate to each situation by the appropriate legal professionals and/or consultants selected by the person. Any references or links to information or to particular organizations or references are provided as a courtesy and convenience, and are not intended to constitute any endorsement of the linked materials or the referenced organizations or materials by the author or publisher. The content and views on such links and of such organizations are solely their own and do not necessarily reflect those of the author or publisher. The author of this publication, Diane L. Darvey, prepared this publication on her own behalf, not as a representative of the National Association of Chain Drug Stores (NACDS). NACDS did not review or approve this publication, and its contents do not necessarily represent the views of NACDS.

Table of Contents

Learning Objectives
Introduction
Role of Laws and Regulations
Role of Pharmacy Professional Practice Standards and Ethical Principles
Violations of Pharmacy Laws and Regulations
Summary
Self-Assessment Questions
Appendix 1-1. Code of Ethics: Pharmacy Associations
Appendix 1-2. Code of Ethics for Pharmacy Technicians: American Association of Pharmacy Technicians (AAPT)

Learning Objectives
Introduction
Federal Laws and Rules or Regulations
State Laws and Rules or Regulations
Role of State Boards of Pharmacy
Summary
References
Self-Assessment Questions

Learning Objectives
Introduction
Food, Drug, and Cosmetic Act: Purpose, History, and Enforcement
Poison Prevention Packaging Act
Omnibus Budget Reconciliation Act of 1990
Medicare Modernization Act of 2003
Summary
References
Self-Assessment Questions

Learning Objectives

Chapter 1

U.S. Legal and Regulatory System

Chapter Outline

Learning Objectives
Introduction
Role of Laws and Regulations
Role of Pharmacy Professional Practice Standards and Ethical Principles
Violations of Pharmacy Laws and Regulations
Summary
Self-Assessment Questions
Appendix 1-1. Code of Ethics: Pharmacy Associations
Appendix 1-2. Code of Ethics for Pharmacy Technicians: American Association of
    Pharmacy Technicians (AAPT)

Learning Objectives

1. Explain key differences between laws/regulations or rules and pharmacy professional practice standards/ethical principles.
2. Identify the function of pharmacy laws and regulations or rules.
3. Discuss how professional standards and ethical principles impact your practice as a pharmacy technician.
4. Compare and contrast the processes required to establish laws, regulations, professional practice standards, and ethical principles.
5. Describe the different legal systems that could be involved for a legal dispute or a violation of a pharmacy law and/or regulation.

Introduction

As part of your education and training to become a pharmacy technician, you will learn how extensively pharmacy is governed by laws and rules or regulations and other requirements, such as pharmacy professional practice standards and ethical principles. You may ask: "Why is there so much oversight?" Perhaps the most obvious reasons are the roles and responsibilities that pharmacists have in overseeing the provision of medications to nearly every member of society—whether by dispensing prescriptions; providing drug information to physicians, nurses, and other health care practitioners; counseling and assisting patients with understanding their drug therapy; or assisting patients with selecting the appropriate over-the-counter medications. Pharmacists are responsible for the delivery of medications and medication or drug therapy-related services in many settings, including community pharmacies, hospitals, long-term care facilities, and other health care sites where prescription medications are dispensed.

Legal requirements, ethical guidelines, and professional practice standards for pharmacy each serve a necessary purpose. They have been developed over many years in order to guide the safe and effective delivery of medications to patients. The oversight for pharmacy practice comes from a variety of sources (**Box 1-1**). Laws and regulations provide governmental oversight of pharmacy practice, including pharmacists and pharmacy technicians. For instance, in order to practice pharmacy, a pharmacist must have a current valid state pharmacy license for each state in which he or she practices. Similarly, many states now have laws or regulations that require pharmacy technicians to be licensed or registered and meet other requirements, such as specific training and education and criminal history background checks.

In contrast, professional practice standards and ethical principles come from different sources such as professional pharmacy organizations. These guidelines and principles provide pharmacists with guidance on delivering pharmacy services to patients so that they meet the expectations of their peers. For example, professional practice standards could assist pharmacists with dispensing medications to patients with particular diseases such as diabetes or high blood pressure.

Box 1-1
Sources of Oversight and Standards for Pharmacy Practice

- Federal laws and regulations
- State laws and regulations
- Professional practice standards
- Ethical principles
- Case law

In dispensing such prescription medications, professional practice standards would guide pharmacists in consulting with the patient's prescriber about recommended medications and avoiding potential drug–drug interactions with other drugs that were prescribed for the patient. Practice standards also guide pharmacists when providing patients with information on how to take their medications properly—according to their doctor's prescription and avoiding drug interactions with over-the-counter drugs.

Ethical principles work in conjunction with the professional practice standards. In simple terms, ethical principles provide guidance for acting in an ethical manner. For example, ethical principles include important matters such as providing services with honesty and integrity, recognizing patient dignity, and obeying laws and regulations applicable to providing pharmacy services. Ethical principles provide a fundamental framework for interacting with the patient—showing care and compassion and maintaining the proper degree of patient privacy about the patient's medical conditions, drug treatment, and other private patient information.

Pharmacy technicians work in a health care field with one of the most highly regarded health care professionals. Nearly every year, health care providers—including pharmacists—are ranked near or at the top among professionals for honesty and integrity in public opinion polls. The polls also consistently rank pharmacists as one of the most trusted professionals.

Although pharmacy technicians may consider legal issues somewhat remote to their day-to-day responsibilities, the opposite is true. Legal requirements apply to nearly all of the pharmacists' professional actions as well as the duties and responsibilities performed by pharmacy technicians. Because pharmacy technicians must comply with the applicable laws and regulations, pharmacy technicians need to know and understand that they work in a field that is subject to numerous laws and regulations. The purpose of this book is to guide you through understanding the legal and regulatory environment applicable to the practice of pharmacy.

Role of Laws and Regulations

Laws and regulations govern virtually all aspects of the practice of pharmacy. They establish permitted and prohibited conduct for pharmacists, pharmacies, and pharmacy technicians. They set the criteria that a pharmacy must satisfy to be licensed by a state and also the criteria that pharmacists must meet to be licensed in a state. They set the requirements that pharmacy technicians must meet to become registered or licensed in a state. The laws and regulations establish the pharmacist's responsibilities for operating a pharmacy, dispensing prescription medications, and providing other pharmacist services such as counseling patients about their medications. They establish the requirements for information that must be on the prescription label, such as the name and quantity of the prescribed medication, directions for use, and other information. State laws and regulations applicable to pharmacy technicians may cover what they are permitted to do; prohibited conduct; and requirements to work as a pharmacy technician, such as registration or licensure and requirements to perform responsibilities under the supervision of a pharmacist.

 # Key Point

Laws and regulations govern virtually all aspects of the practice of pharmacy.

Laws (also known as statutes) have primary authority over regulations. However, both have legal effect over the practice of pharmacy, pharmacists, pharmacy technicians, and pharmacies. In general terms, laws are enacted by the U.S. Congress or by a state legislature, and agencies adopt rules that interpret the laws in more details. State laws and regulations vary from state to state. Every U.S. state, territory, and the District of Columbia has its own laws and regulations governing pharmacy practice. While they may have similarities, they differ in many respects. One of these differences is how pharmacy technicians are regulated. These similarities and differences will be covered in greater detail in Chapter 6 (**Box 1-2**).

States have the authority to regulate the practice of pharmacy. However, federal laws and regulations also have an effect on various parts of pharmacy practice. Examples include laws that are applicable to all health care providers (e.g., the Medicare and Medicaid laws), laws directed at medications (e.g., the Federal Food, Drug, and Cosmetic Act), and laws directed at specific types of drugs (e.g., the federal Controlled Substances Act). As a special note, there are federal employers of pharmacists such as the U.S. Public Health Services and the armed services. Federal laws will be discussed in more detail in Chapter 3.

Although states have the primary authority to regulate pharmacy practice, one particular federal law significantly affects pharmacy practice. The federal Omnibus Budget Reconciliation Act of 1990 (commonly called "OBRA 90") was the first federal law to address the standards of practice for pharmacists. OBRA '90 requires

---

Box 1-2
Pharmacy Laws and Regulations or Rules

- Establish required, permitted, and prohibited conduct
- Provide for discipline and penalties for violations
- Vary from state to state
- Control pharmacy practice, licensure, and discipline

that pharmacists provide certain patient services as a condition of reimbursement when dispensing prescriptions to Medicaid patients. Because the states regulate the practice of pharmacy, the federal legislation takes an indirect approach by requiring that pharmacists perform certain patient care functions as a condition of reimbursement. OBRA '90 will be discussed in Chapter 3.

Laws and regulations are derived by different means. Enacting state or federal laws involves the state or federal legislature, respectively. State legislatures are comprised of two bodies, generally known as the House and Senate, although they may have other names depending on the state. State legislation must be passed by both the House and Senate and then become law through being signed by the Governor or otherwise allowed under the state law. However, laws passed by state legislatures may not become law through different actions. For instance, the state's Governor may veto legislation. If vetoed, the bill would not become law. If the bill is not signed by the Governor, it may become law if state laws allow it. Federal legislation must be approved by both the U.S. House of Representatives and the U.S. Senate to be eligible to become law; as with the states, the legislation then goes to the President for approval or veto. The state and federal processes for enacting legislation into laws are discussed in Chapter 2.

Regulations or rules, on the other hand, are issued by state administrative agencies or regulatory bodies pursuant to the authority granted to them by the laws or statutes. Most state Boards of Pharmacy are administrative agencies with authority to propose and adopt regulations to further implement pharmacy laws. For example, a state law that gives the Board of Pharmacy authority to regulate and license or register pharmacy technicians would also usually permit the Board of Pharmacy to adopt rules or regulations with more detailed requirements for pharmacy technician licensure or registration. These detailed regulatory requirements may include specific education and training, age requirements, and basic education level such as a high school degree.

 ## Key Point

Most state Boards of Pharmacy are administrative agencies with authority to propose and adopt regulations to further implement pharmacy laws.

The regulatory process for a Board of Pharmacy to adopt regulations varies from state to state, but there are a number of basic similarities. In general, the Board is required to issue a formal public notice of the proposed regulation. Next, the Board is required in most instances to allow the public (e.g., pharmacists and other interested persons) to send comments to the Board if they have concerns or questions. In addition, the Board may be required to hold a public hearing to receive comments in person. Thereafter, several options exist depending on the state laws. For example, the proposed regulation may be approved as initially proposed and adopted as a final regulation. Alternatively, the proposed regulation may be amended in response to comments received and reissued as a revised regulation. At the federal level, the process is generally similar. Regulations proposed by a federal regulatory agency are published for public comment. Once a regulation becomes effective by meeting the state or federal requirements for the approval process, it will be published in the state administrative code or Code of Federal Regulations as a final regulation.

Although the states have primary authority to license and regulate the practice of pharmacy, federal laws and regulations have authority over matters that affect pharmacy practice by governing how drugs are manufactured, distributed, and handled. For example, the federal Food and Drug Administration (FDA) regulates drugs that are available for use in the United States from manufacturing, distribution, labeling, and marketing to the determination of whether drugs are safe and effective for use in the United States. The federal Drug Enforcement Administration (DEA) regulates the subset of drugs called "controlled substances," which includes drugs such as narcotics and sleeping medications.

Pharmacy practice is affected by both state and federal laws. As a general rule, when the state and federal laws have different requirements, the more stringent law must be followed. If federal law is less strict than state law, the stricter state law would be followed and vice versa. For example, if a federal law has specific requirements for dispensing controlled substances, and a state pharmacy law has added stricter requirements, the additional stricter state law requirement would be followed in addition to the federal requirements.

Role of Pharmacy Professional Practice Standards and Ethical Principles

The practice of pharmacy is also affected by professional practice standards and ethical principles. Once a pharmacist is educated and licensed to practice pharmacy, the practice standards and ethical principles provide further guidance for pharmacists in the delivery of pharmacy services. Pharmacy is not unique in having professional practice standards and ethical principles. Other health care professionals, including physicians, dentists, and nurses, have practice standards and ethical guidelines.

Professional Practice Standards

Professional practice standards serve as guidelines for pharmacists to use with professional judgment in determining how to act in particular situations. Practice standards are not laws or regulations. They serve an important role in pharmacy and the practice of other health care professionals by assisting providers with decision-making processes such as recommendations for treatment of a patient and provision of pharmacy services and other health care services.

 # Key Point

Professional practice standards serve as guidelines for pharmacists to use with professional judgment in determining how to act in particular situations.

The definitions of the "practice of pharmacy" and "pharmacist care" are helpful in understanding professional practice standards because they describe the scope of pharmacy practice. These definitions show that the practice of pharmacy involves a number of different pharmacist responsibilities. Professional practice standards may relate to these areas of the practice of pharmacy. The Model Rules of the National Association of Boards of Pharmacy (NABP) define the practice of pharmacy and "pharmacist care" as shown below.

The "Practice of Pharmacy" means the interpretation, evaluation, and implementation of medical orders; the dispensing of prescription drug orders; participation in drug and device selection; drug administration; drug regimen reviews; the practice of telepharmacy within and across state lines; drug or drug-related research; the provision of patient counseling and the provision of those acts or services necessary to provide pharmaceutical care in all areas of patient care, including primary care and collaborative pharmacy practice; and the responsibility for compounding and labeling of drugs and devices (except labeling by a manufacturer, repackager, or distributor of non-prescription drugs and commercially packaged legend drugs and devices), proper and safe storage of drugs and devices, and maintenance of proper records for them. (See NABP Model Rules at http://www.nabp.net.)

"Pharmacist Care" is the provision by a Pharmacist of Medication Therapy Management Services, with or without the Dispensing of Drugs or Devices, intended to achieve outcomes related to the cure or prevention of a disease, elimination or reduction of a patient's symptoms, or arresting or slowing of a disease process, as defined in the Rules of the Board. (See NABP Model Rules at http://www.nabp.net.)

Pharmacy practice standards come from a variety of sources; however, they are usually developed by professional pharmacy organizations through a panel of pharmacists with input from leaders of the profession. Pharmacy practice standards have been developed by a number of national pharmacy organizations. For example, two such organizations, the American Pharmacists Association (APhA) and the American Association of Colleges of Pharmacy (AACP), worked together to create the APhA/AACP Standards of Practice of the Profession of Pharmacy. The national professional association for health-system pharmacists, the American Society of Health-System Pharmacists (ASHP), also developed professional standards for pharmacists.

 # Key Point

Pharmacy practice standards are usually developed by professional pharmacy organizations through a panel of pharmacists with input from leaders of the profession.

Although professional practice standards are not laws or regulations developed by legislatures or regulatory agencies, they have a significant impact on pharmacy practice. They may guide the pharmacist's consultation with the patient's physician. For example, if a pharmacist is concerned about a potential drug–drug interaction with the patient's prescribed medication, professional standards may provide guidance to the pharmacist for evaluating the potential drug interaction and contacting the prescriber to recommend an alternate medication for the patient.

Ethical Principles

Ethical principles, on the other hand, guide the performance of professional responsibilities within an ethical and moral framework. They guide pharmacists' and pharmacy technicians' interactions and relationships with patients and other health care professionals to conform to society's ethical values. In simple terms, acting according to ethical principles means doing the "right thing" and acting in consideration of the patient. Following ethical principles also includes a number of other considerations such as complying with the applicable laws and regulations, promoting high professional standards in providing care to patients, maintaining professional competency, and respecting patient privacy and confidentiality. Pharmacy technicians also need to adhere to ethical principles. For example, pharmacy technicians become aware of confidential patient information. Ethical principles (as well as privacy laws and regulations) require respect for the patient's privacy and preventing inappropriate disclosure of a patient's private information. ASHP and APhA have both developed their own Code of Ethics for Pharmacists (see **Appendix 1-1**). The American Association of Pharmacy Technicians (AAPT) has developed a Code of Ethics for Pharmacy Technicians (see **Appendix 1-2**).

⚜ **Key Point**

Ethical principles guide the performance of professional responsibilities within an ethical and moral framework.

Violations of Pharmacy Laws and Regulations

There are different legal systems where violations of pharmacy laws and regulations may be addressed: a disciplinary action with an administrative hearing before the state Board of Pharmacy, a civil court proceeding, and a criminal court proceeding. Of these, violations of pharmacy laws and regulations are normally considered and determined by the state Board of Pharmacy as disciplinary actions. However, violations of pharmacy laws and regulations may be a part of other legal proceedings.

These are the general steps involved with a Board of Pharmacy disciplinary matter; however, the process may vary from state to state. A disciplinary action against a pharmacist, pharmacy technician, or pharmacy usually starts with a complaint being received by the Board of Pharmacy or where a violation is found during a Board of Pharmacy inspection. The Board of Pharmacy will conduct an investigation to determine the circumstances, appropriate Board action, and will notify the pharmacy, pharmacy technician, and/or pharmacist of the violation. Depending on the Board's determination, the Board may dismiss the matter without a Board hearing, or may recommend that the person or pharmacy agree to take corrective actions. If the disciplinary action comes before the Board of Pharmacy for a hearing, the Board will consider the violation and circumstances to determine the type of penalties to be applied, if any. Possible penalties include monetary fines and temporary or permanent loss of the license or registration. For instance, a law or regulation may not permit a pharmacy technician to perform certain responsibilities or duties or only allow the technician to perform them if the individual is a Certified Pharmacy Technician. A pharmacy technician that violates the law or regulation would receive a notice of a violation, and a Board hearing would usually be held. At the hearing, the facts would be discussed and the pharmacy technician would be permitted to provide information regarding the matter to the Board such as explaining the circumstances. A technician may decide to have legal representation (i.e., an attorney) at the disciplinary hearing. The hearing is a legal process to resolve the violation and decide whether a penalty is appropriate. The same general process would apply to violations issued by a Board of Pharmacy against a pharmacist or pharmacy. This is a general discussion of the process as the particular process may vary considerably depending on the state.

Violations of pharmacy laws and regulations may also be a part of a civil lawsuit. This is a general discussion because these lawsuits are complicated in many instances. An example is a lawsuit for professional negligence (also called a medical malpractice case). These types of lawsuits generally involve a patient claiming injury as a result of medical treatment. For instance, a patient could claim that he or she was injured as a result of a prescription being filled incorrectly and may use the violation of the pharmacy law or regulation as part of the professional negligence case. When such disputes arise, the civil court system operates to resolve them through lawsuits with juries to determine if the defendant was or was not negligent. In some instances, the parties to the cases may decide to resolve the matter through an alternative dispute resolution process such as arbitration or mediation. If the case goes to trial, the facts and circumstances will be considered by the jury to determine if the defendant or defendants were at fault in causing the patient's injuries.

In some matters, although very rare, the violations of pharmacy laws or regulations may be criminal in nature; criminal penalties would be handled in the criminal courts. Although rare, this could occur when the charges involve violations of criminal laws and the state or federal prosecutor or district attorney decides to bring criminal charges. In general, criminal violations involve wrongful conduct that was intentional.

Summary

The pharmacy profession is extensively regulated by laws and regulations that govern virtually every aspect of the practice of pharmacy such as pharmacist and pharmacy licensure requirements, scope of pharmacist practice, prescription dispensing requirements, use of pharmacy technicians, prohibited conduct, and disciplinary actions. Although pharmacy laws and regulations have general similarities, the specific requirements vary from state to state. Violations of pharmacy laws and regulations, including violations by pharmacy technicians, are generally handled by the state Board of Pharmacy.

Laws and regulations are derived by different means. State legislatures enact laws, whereas state administrative agencies such as state Boards of Pharmacy adopt regulations. Many states have laws specifically applicable to pharmacy technicians, including requirements for registration or licensure and permitted duties. Because laws and regulations vary from state to state, pharmacy technicians should be knowledgeable about the ones operating in their specific state. The pharmacy profession is also subject to pharmacy professional practice standards and ethical principles. Practice standards provide guidelines for the delivery of pharmacy services. Ethical principles guide the performance of pharmacy care within an ethical and moral framework.

Self-Assessment Questions

1. What are three sources of oversight and standards for pharmacy practice?
2. What federal agency regulates the subset of drugs called "controlled substances," which includes drugs such as narcotics and sleeping medications?
3. What is a federal law that affects pharmacy practice for pharmacists?
4. What organizations have developed professional practice standards for pharmacy?
5. What regulatory body issues a notice of violation if there is a violation of a pharmacy law or regulation?

Appendix 1-1. Code of Ethics: Pharmacy Associations

American Pharmaceutical Association Code of Ethics for Pharmacists (APhA)

(Endorsed by the American Society for Health-System Pharmacists)

Preamble

Pharmacists are health professionals who assist individuals in making the best use of medications. This Code, prepared and supported by pharmacists, is intended to state publicly the principles that form the fundamental basis of the roles and responsibilities of pharmacists. These principles, based on moral obligations and virtues, are established to guide pharmacists in relationships with patients, health professionals, and society.

I.   **A pharmacist respects the covenantal relationship between the patient and pharmacist.**

Considering the patient–pharmacist relationship as a covenant means that a pharmacist has moral obligations in response to the gift of trust received from society. In return for this gift, a pharmacist promises to help individuals achieve optimum benefit from their medications, to be committed to their welfare, and to maintain their trust.

II. **A pharmacist promotes the good of every patient in a caring, compassionate, and confidential manner.**

A pharmacist places concern for the well-being of the patient at the center of professional practice. In doing so, a pharmacist considers needs stated by the patient as well as those defined by health science. A pharmacist is dedicated to protecting the dignity of the patient. With a caring attitude and a compassionate spirit, a pharmacist focuses on serving the patient in a private and confidential manner.

III. **A pharmacist respects the autonomy and dignity of each patient.**

A pharmacist promotes the right of self-determination and recognizes individual self-worth by encouraging patients to participate in decisions about their health. A pharmacist communicates with patients in terms that are understandable. In all cases, a pharmacist respects personal and cultural differences among patients.

IV.   A pharmacist acts with honesty and integrity in professional relationships.

A pharmacist has a duty to tell the truth and to act with conviction of conscience. A pharmacist avoids discriminatory practices, behavior, or work conditions that impair professional judgment, and actions that compromise dedication to the best interests of patients.

V.   A pharmacist maintains professional competence.

A pharmacist has a duty to maintain knowledge and abilities as new medications, devices, and technologies become available and as health information advances.

VI.   A pharmacist respects the values and abilities of colleagues and other health professionals.

When appropriate, a pharmacist asks for the consultation of colleagues or other health professionals or refers the patient. A pharmacist acknowledges that colleagues and other health professionals may differ in the beliefs and values they apply to the care of the patient.

VII.   A pharmacist serves individual, community, and societal needs.

The primary obligation of a pharmacist is to individual patients. However, the obligations of a pharmacist may at times extend beyond the individual to the community and society. In these situations, the pharmacist recognizes the responsibilities that accompany these obligations and acts accordingly.

VIII. A pharmacist seeks justice in the distribution of health resources.

When health resources are allocated, a pharmacist is fair and equitable, balancing the needs of patients and society.

Appendix 1-2. Code of Ethics for Pharmacy Technicians: American Association of Pharmacy Technicians (AAPT)

Code of Ethics for Pharmacy Technicians

Preamble

Pharmacy Technicians are healthcare professionals who assist pharmacists in providing the best possible care for patients. The principles of this code, which apply to pharmacy technicians working in any and all settings, are based on the application and support of the moral obligations that guide the pharmacy profession in relationships with patients, healthcare professionals and society.

Principles

▶ A pharmacy technician's first consideration is to ensure the health and safety of the patient, and to use knowledge and skills to the best of his/her ability in serving patients.

▶ A pharmacy technician supports and promotes honesty and integrity in the profession, which includes a duty to observe the law, maintain the highest moral and ethical conduct at all times and uphold the ethical principles of the profession.

▶ A pharmacy technician assists and supports the pharmacists in the safe and efficacious and cost effective distribution of health services and healthcare resources.

▶ A pharmacy technician respects and values the abilities of pharmacists, colleagues and other healthcare professionals.

▶ A pharmacy technician maintains competency in his/her practice and continually enhances his/her professional knowledge and expertise.

▶ A pharmacy technician respects and supports the patient's individuality, dignity, and confidentiality.

▶ A pharmacy technician respects the confidentiality of a patient's records and discloses pertinent information only with proper authorization.

▶ A pharmacy technician never assists in dispensing, promoting or distribution of medication or medical devices that are not of good quality or do not meet the standards required by law.

▶ A pharmacy technician does not engage in any activity that will discredit the profession, and will expose, without fear or favor, illegal or unethical conduct of the profession.

▶ A pharmacy technician associates with and engages in the support of organizations, which promote the profession of pharmacy through the utilization and enhancement of pharmacy technicians.

Chapter 2

Development of Laws and Rules or Regulations

Chapter Outline

Learning Objectives

1. Identify the different branches of government and their roles.
2. Describe the process that bills must undergo to become law.
3. Discuss the process for creation of rules or regulations.
4. Identify the primary differences between federal and state legislatures.
5. Discuss the role and authority of state Boards of Pharmacy and how this impacts you as a pharmacy technician.

Introduction

The goal of this chapter is to help you understand how laws and regulations are made—how a bill becomes a law and how proposed rules or regulations become adopted final rules or regulations. *Legislative process* is the term that is commonly used to describe the means by which a proposed bill or legislation becomes a law (also called a *statute*). The process of creating rules or regulations is commonly called the *regulatory or rulemaking process*. This chapter will discuss the federal and state legislative and regulatory processes and the role of the state Board of Pharmacy in creating regulations governing the practice of pharmacy.

Branches of Government

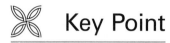 Key Point

Federal and state governments are comprised of three branches: legislative, executive, and judicial.

Both the federal and state governments are comprised of three branches: legislative, executive, and judicial. Each of these branches has a different governmental role. Legislatures make laws or statutes by introducing and enacting legislation. The executive branch enforces the laws, and the judicial branch interprets laws (**Table 2-1**).

The state government, as at the national level, is composed of three branches. The legislative branch creates laws, the executive branch carries out the laws, and the judicial branch interprets the laws (**Table 2-2**).

Table 2-1
Branches of the U.S. Government

Branches	Components	Function
Legislative	U.S. Congress • Senate • House of Representatives	Makes laws
Executive	President of the United States Vice President of the United States Cabinet Executive agencies	Enforces laws
Judicial	U.S. Supreme Court Federal courts	Interprets laws and U.S. Constitution

Table 2-2
Branches of State Government

Branches	Components	Function
Legislative	State Congress • Senate • House of Representatives	Makes laws
Executive	Governor Executives Executive agencies	Enforces state laws
Judicial	State court system	Interprets state laws

Administrative Agencies

Administrative agencies (also known as regulatory agencies) are part of the executive branch. The actions of administrative agencies include proposing and adopting rules (also called regulations) as well as enforcing rules and regulations through administrative actions such as disciplinary investigations, citations, hearings, and other administrative actions. There are many state and federal administrative agencies. Examples of federal agencies include the Food and Drug Administration (FDA), which enforces the Food, Drug, and Cosmetic Act and issues regulations, and the Drug Enforcement Administration (DEA), which regulates the use of drugs designated as controlled substances.

 # Key Point

The actions of administrative agencies include proposing and adopting rules (also called regulations) as well as enforcing rules through administrative actions such as disciplinary investigations, citations, hearings, and other administrative actions.

The state Board of Pharmacy is the state administrative agency that usually oversees pharmacies, pharmacists, pharmacy technicians, and other aspects of the practice of pharmacy. (The state Board of Pharmacy will be discussed in more detail at the end of this chapter.) States also may have drug enforcement agencies similar to the federal DEA regulating the use and dispensing of drugs that are designated as controlled substance drugs. State Boards of Pharmacy also regulate the distribution and dispensing of controlled substances by pharmacies.

 # Key Point

The state Board of Pharmacy is the state administrative agency that oversees pharmacies, pharmacists, pharmacy technicians, and other aspects of the practice of pharmacy.

Role of Laws

Laws affect many aspects of society, including pharmacy. Reasons for laws come from many sources such as interest groups that approach legislators with a particular concern or problem. They also come from legislators and agencies that become aware of issues to be addressed. Generally, this leads to a large number of bills being introduced each year in both the U.S. Congress and in the state legislatures. However, of the many bills introduced each year, only a small number are actually enacted and become law. The primary reasons are the complexity of the legislative process and the difficulty in gathering the number of votes necessary for a bill to be passed by both the House and the Senate.

Laws (also called statutes) are usually broad in scope and express the general intent of the legislation. For instance, a state may decide that pharmacy technicians must be licensed or registered and meet certain educational requirements to become licensed or registered in a particular state. The laws usually do not provide all of the details needed to implement the law. In this example, the law may not provide details of how registration or licensure is handled by the Board of Pharmacy and the particular requirements for registration or licensure. This is where the regulatory process steps in. The appropriate state agency, in this instance the state Board of Pharmacy, would have the authority to issue rules or regulations in response to the law to establish the details for registration or licensure and other pharmacy technician requirements.

Federal Laws and Rules or Regulations

The U.S. Congress has a number of powers such as passing federal laws, overseeing federal agencies, appointing judges to the federal courts (e.g., U.S. Supreme Court and federal district courts), and other responsibilities. The U.S. Constitution gives Congress its legislative powers and establishes that Congress is comprised of the Senate and House of Representatives. The Constitution also provides Congress with the authority to make all laws that are "necessary and proper" for its responsibilities. The Tenth Amendment to the U.S. Constitution gives states the authority to legislate in areas that are not exclusively reserved to the U.S. Congress by the U.S. Constitution. Because many areas are not reserved exclusively to the Congress, states generally have wide legislative authority. Federal and state laws have different applications. Federal laws cover the United States, and state laws apply to each respective state.

 Key Point

The U.S. Congress has power to make federal laws, oversee federal agencies, and make judicial appointments and other responsibilities.

Federal Legislative Process

Creating a federal law is a complicated, lengthy process. It generally begins when a member of Congress, a Senator, or a Representative "introduces" legislation. **Table 2-3** shows the major steps.

The legislation is introduced into either the Senate or the House depending on whether the legislator is a Senator or a Representative. For example, if legis-

Table 2-3
Federal Legislative Process

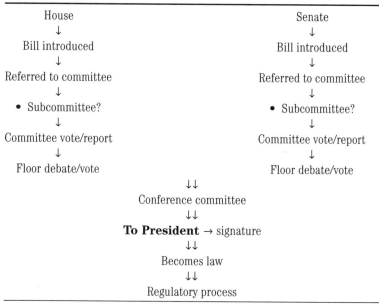

House	Senate
↓	↓
Bill introduced	Bill introduced
↓	↓
Referred to committee	Referred to committee
↓	↓
• Subcommittee?	• Subcommittee?
↓	↓
Committee vote/report	Committee vote/report
↓	↓
Floor debate/vote	Floor debate/vote

↓↓
Conference committee
↓↓
To President → signature
↓↓
Becomes law
↓↓
Regulatory process

lation is sponsored by a Senator, it will be introduced into the Senate and given a number with an "S" in front of the number (e.g., S. 500, meaning Senate bill number 500). Similarly, bills sponsored by a Representative start in the House of Representatives and usually have a preceding "H.R." for House of Representatives (e.g., H.R. 500). The usual steps in the process are 1) bill introduction; 2) referral to the appropriate committee, which may refer the bill to a subcommittee of that committee; and 3) consideration by the committee (and by the subcommittee if selected) with a public hearing. At a public hearing, the committee hears witnesses with opinions on the bill. A bill must pass favorably out of a committee (and any subcommittee) to proceed. The committee may "mark up" the bill with changes (amendments). If voted favorably out of the committee and subcommittee, the bill may be considered, debated, and voted on the "floor" of the House or Senate depending on where it was introduced. Because bills must be passed by both the Senate and House before being eligible for signature by the President, a similar process would be followed in either the House or Senate depending on where the bill started. However, the bill could never come up for a vote in the committee and could "die" without a vote; or if passed out of the committee, it may not be considered by the House or Senate. If the bill is passed by the House or Senate, it would then go to the other chamber for a vote. Once the bill passes both the House and Senate, the language may differ. If there are differences, the bill goes to a "conference committee" with members of the House and Senate to work out the differences so that the House and Senate versions of the bill would be the same. Roadblocks to passage may occur such as the conference committee not meeting or not resolving the differences. If the differences between the House and Senate versions are resolved, the bill would likely need to go back to both the House and Senate for another vote. If the identical bill passes both the House and Senate, it is considered enrolled. It is sent to the President for signature. The President has options:

▶ Sign the bill into law.
▶ Pocket veto the bill at the end of the Congressional session.
▶ Let it become law without signing it.
▶ Veto the bill and return it to Congress.

If the President vetoes the bill, Congress can override the Presidential veto with a 2/3 vote in both the House and Senate.

As you can see, the legislative process is long and arduous, making it very difficult for legislation to be enacted into law. This difficult process may serve a purpose ensuring that laws enacted represent a consensus of all the various stakeholders that may be affected by the law.

Once a law is enacted, the final step is to publish the law in the appropriate section of the United States Code. The U.S. Code is the official record of all the federal laws.

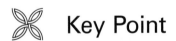 **Key Point**

The U.S. Code is the official record of all the federal laws.

Federal Regulatory Process

Once a bill becomes law, implementation often requires regulations because laws usually lack details for their implementation and use. For instance, federal law requires prescription drugs to be manufactured safely, and the federal Food and Drug Administration (FDA) has adopted regulations providing specific regulatory requirements for drug manufacturers. The FDA also enforces the federal laws and adopts regulations governing drug manufacturers.

There are more than 50 federal regulatory agencies. In addition to the FDA, other examples that you may be familiar with include the Environmental Protection Agency (EPA) and the Drug Enforcement Administration (DEA), which is part of the U.S. Department of Justice.

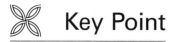 # Key Point

There are more than 50 federal regulatory agencies.

The federal regulatory process is governed by the Federal Register Act[1] and the Administrative Procedures Act (APA).[2] The Federal Register Act sets the requirements for rules published in the *Code of Federal Regulations*. The Administrative Procedures Act establishes the steps that federal agencies must follow as they adopt rules and regulations to implement and enforce laws. For example, federal agencies are required to publish the rule and allow interested parties such as the public or associations representing different groups to comment on the rule. The comments may include any concerns, objections, or changes (i.e., amendments) they recommend. The Administrative Procedures Act describes the allowed scope of the rules such as explaining the law and the procedures to be followed to comply with the law. It explains the rulemaking purpose as being "essentially legislative in nature" because the rules establish policy (**Box 2-1**).

The regulatory rulemaking process starts with a federal agency determining that a regulation is needed or required. The next steps are the agency's preparation of the proposed rule followed by publication of the proposed rule in the *Federal Register*, making it available for public review and opportunity to comment back to the agency on the proposed rule. In some instances, the agency also holds a public hearing. The publication in the *Federal Register* is the *official* notice of the agency's intent to adopt a new rule or amend (change) an existing rule. The published notice also informs the public of the deadline date by which comments are due and where to send comments, and if a hearing is held, the date, time, and location on the hearing.

Box 2-1
Federal Regulatory Process

Agency determination or required to issue rule
↓
Preparation of proposed rule
↓
Notice of publication of proposed rule
↓
Public comment period
↓
Preparation of final rule
↓
Publication of final rule

The public's comments may be in favor of or against the proposed rules, and may ask the agency to change the proposed rule. Federal agencies often receive a large number of comments. The agency may or may not revise the rule in response to the comments. If the proposed rule is revised, the agency would publish the text of the revised proposed rule in the *Federal Register*. However, the agency may republish the proposed rule without changes and provide the effective date of the new rule. Once a rule has been published as a final rule in the *Federal Register*, it is published in the *Code of Federal Regulations (CFR)*. The *CFR* is the *official* book of adopted federal rules.

Another federal law makes tracking the large number of federal proposed regulations easier. The Regulatory Flexibility Act[3] requires that federal agencies consider a number of factors such as the economic effect of the regulation on small businesses and to add oversight to the regulatory process. Part of the process requires federal agencies to publish their planned upcoming regulatory activities in the *Federal Register*. Tracking federal regulations has also been made easier with the Internet. The federal government has a website for information on the *Federal Register* rules at http://www.gpoaccess.gov/fr/index.html.

State Laws and Rules or Regulations

State Laws

The lawmaking process in the states mirrors the federal process in most respects. However, there are differences because each state has authority to determine the details of their legislative process. Some differences between federal and state legislatures are the duration of the legislative session and the types of legislative committees and processes. The U.S. Congress is in session each year for most of the year. However, in some states the legislative session lasts for only a few months each year, and some states have legislative sessions every other year instead of yearly. There are also likely to be differences in the types of legislative committees, reports prepared by the legislative committees, and the legislative hearings. Federally, legislation tends to be accompanied by more comprehensive committee reports that detail the intent of Congress and may involve many more hearings, whereas states may have different procedures and types of reports that accompany the legislation.

 Key Point

The primary differences between federal and state legislatures are the duration of the legislative session, the frequency, and the types of legislative committees and processes.

There are some similarities between the states and the U.S. Congress. As with the federal government, states have three branches of government consisting of the state legislature, the executive branch, and the judicial branch. Similarly, state legislatures are comprised of two chambers, the House and the Senate. However, states may use different names. For instance, in some states, the House may be called the House of Representatives and in others called the House of Delegates. The members of the state Senate (Senators) are elected by the state's residents as are the members of the state's House (whether Representatives or Delegates). Table 2-2 illustrates the branches of state government and their functions.

The starting process for creating a state law, as at the federal level, occurs when a member of the state legislature proposes a bill or legislation and then sponsors it for introduction in the respective chamber. In other ways, the legislative process is similar. As in the U.S. Congress, a bill would be sent to the appropriate committee for consideration, and must be heard and successfully voted on by both the House and Senate in a state. If voted on successfully by both the House and Senate, the bill must also go to the Governor for consideration where it may be signed or vetoed or have no action taken.

State Regulations

The state rulemaking process has many similarities to the federal process. States have a number of regulatory administrative agencies that are empowered to adopt rules and regulations pursuant to power granted by state laws. In many states, the state Board of Pharmacy has the power to adopt pharmacy regulations. However, in other states, the state Board of Pharmacy may be part of a larger state agency (such as the Department of Health) that has authority to adopt pharmacy regulations with the involvement of the Board of Pharmacy.

Like the federal system, adopting state regulations is governed by state law. Each state has an Administrative Procedures Act or similar law establishing requirements that the state agencies must follow when proposing and adopting regulations or rules. These requirements generally include giving notice of proposed new or amended rules or regulations through publication in the state's register or other appropriate publication, giving the public a minimum time period to provide comments (usually 30 days or longer), and including notice of hearings where the proposed rules will be discussed. State agencies must also publish the final rules and effective date of the final rules (**Box 2-2**).

In some states, the rules adopted by a state agency are reviewed by a state legislative rule review committee. If an agency's adopted rule is approved through the legislative rule review, it becomes a final adopted rule and becomes effective on a particular date as determined by the agency. The final rule is then published in the state register or similar publication source and placed into the state's official administrative rules.

Box 2-2
State Regulatory Process

State agency (e.g., state Board of Pharmacy)
→ determines need or law requires rule
↓
Preparation of proposed rule
↓
Publication of proposed rule
↓
Public comment period and hearings
↓
Publication of final rule

 Key Point

In some states, the rules adopted by a state agency are reviewed by a state legislative rule review committee.

Role of State Boards of Pharmacy

State Boards of Pharmacy are granted their authority by the state law, which creates the Board and sets out what they are entitled to do. For example, many states are now beginning to license or register pharmacy technicians. For Boards of Pharmacy to have this authority, the states must introduce bills to change the pharmacy laws in order to give this authority to the state Boards of Pharmacy. The process of enacting these laws would follow the legislative process; interested members of the public and the pharmacy community would have the opportunity to comment on the proposed legislation for pharmacy technician licensure or registration.

The primary authority of state pharmacy boards is to regulate the practice of pharmacy in the state. For that reason, the pharmacy laws and regulations are often referred to as the *pharmacy practice laws and regulations*. In some states, the state Boards of Pharmacy may have some authority over certain aspects of the responsibilities of other health care providers. For instance, the state Board may have authority over the dispensing of prescription medications in a physician's office. This additional authority varies greatly from state to state.

Nearly every year, Boards of Pharmacy issue new regulations or modify existing regulations to keep pace with changes in the practice of pharmacy. State Boards of Pharmacy have different sources to provide information on new and proposed regulation changes. Most state Boards of Pharmacy have a website, and newsletters are published routinely to keep pharmacists and pharmacy technicians aware of the pharmacy laws and regulations. The National Association of Boards of Pharmacy maintains a list of contact information for state Boards of Pharmacy at http://www.nabp.net.

Summary

State and federal governments are comprised of three different branches: legislative, executive, and judicial. Each branch has a different governmental role. Legislatures enact laws, the executive branch executes and administers laws, and the judicial branch interprets laws. Administrative agencies, such as the state Boards of Pharmacy, are part of the executive branch with responsibility for adopting regulations and enforcing laws and regulations. The process of enacting laws, whether by the U.S. Congress or a state legislature, is a complex process. The regulatory proposal and adoption process is governed by laws that establish the process for proposal and adopting regulations. This chapter provides general guidelines on the federal and state legislative and regulatory processes. State Boards of Pharmacy provide information on existing pharmacy laws and regulations as well as new regulations proposed by the state Board of Pharmacy through different sources, including websites and newsletters.

References

1. See 44 United States Code Sections 1501-1511.
2. See 5 United States Code 511-599.
3. See 5 United States Code 602.

Self-Assessment Questions

1. What is the role of the legislative branch of both the state and federal government?
2. State governments are composed of what branches of government?
3. Who can introduce federal legislation?
4. The FDA, EPA, and DEA are all examples of what type of federal agency?
5. Pharmacy laws and regulations are also often referred to by what common name?

Chapter 3

Federal Laws and Regulations for Drugs

Chapter Outline

Learning Objectives

1. Match the Food, Drug, and Cosmetic Act and its amendments to their purpose.
2. List and describe the three parts of the Food, Drug, and Cosmetic Act.
3. Discuss the effects of the Kefauver–Harris Amendment on the medication approval process.
4. Describe the need for patient package inserts.
5. List the authority areas and examples of each of the FDA.
6. Identify the types of recalls that may be issued by the FDA.
7. Discuss the impact of the Prescription Drug Marketing Act on the drug distribution system.
8. Identify the three services that pharmacists must provide according to OBRA '90.
9. List counseling points that should be covered, according to OBRA '90, during counseling a patient on a medication.
10. Discuss the changes that the Medicare Modernization Act of 2003 made regarding prescription medications dispensed at a community pharmacy.

Introduction

The goal of this chapter is to describe the various federal laws and regulations that affect prescription drugs, including distribution, manufacturing, control, marketing, and dispensing in the United States. This chapter will discuss the regulation of drugs in the United States, from the development of the Food, Drug, and Cosmetic Act; the Food and Drug Administration; and other federal laws and regulations governing drugs.

Food, Drug, and Cosmetic Act: Purpose, History, and Enforcement

The Food, Drug, and Cosmetic Act of 1938 (FDCA)[1] is the primary federal law controlling prescription drugs in the United States. Another important federal law controlling prescription drugs is the Controlled Substances Act, which will be discussed in Chapter 5. The FDCA regulates manufacturers and distributors of prescription drugs, over-the-counter (OTC) drugs, medical devices, food products, and cosmetics to ensure safety and quality. For instance, the FDCA sets requirements for drug manufacturing and the drug approval process. The law also allows the Food and Drug Administration (FDA) to determine which drugs require a prescription (labeled as *Rx Only*) and which drugs may be purchased directly by a consumer without a prescription (i.e. "over-the-counter" or OTC drugs). Examples of FDA's regulation of food products are requirements for the content of food labels and prohibitions against these labels containing improper claims of health benefits.

The FDCA establishes requirements to ensure that drugs approved for use in the United States are safe, effective, and sold with labeling information that is truthful and not false, misleading, or deceptive. The FDCA contains comprehensive requirements for drugs distributed in the United States. These include requirements for the manufacturing, distribution, labeling, and marketing of drugs and restrictions on importation of drugs into the United States from other countries. For example, drugs cannot be distributed or sold in the United States unless they 1) have met the requirements for evaluation and testing, 2) received prior approval from the FDA, 3) meet FDCA manufacturing requirements, and 4) are shown to be safe and effective. Drugs must be sold with FDA-approved labeling that provides adequate directions for their use.

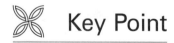 **Key Point**

The FDCA establishes requirements to ensure that drugs approved for use in the United States are safe and effective.

Two provisions through which FDA enforces the FDCA are prohibitions against the distribution of drugs that are *adulterated* or *misbranded*. A drug product would be considered adulterated if the strength, purity, or quality is below the recognized standards. One example is a drug that does not contain the correct drug or contains the incorrect amount of the drug or was manufactured improperly. A drug product may be found misbranded for a number of reasons. For example, a drug would be misbranded if the drug's label does not contain the drug's proper (i.e., established) name and strength, required directions for use, required warnings, or if the drug packaging does not meet the requirement of the Poison Prevention Packaging Act.

History

As early as the mid-1800s, Congress began legislative efforts to control the quality of drugs in the United States. The Drug Importation Act of 1848 allowed U.S. Customs to stop importation of adulterated drugs from other countries into the United States. Concerns about public health and safety from unsafe and poorly labeled drug products led Congress to enact the first law to prohibit distribution of adulterated and misbranded drugs and food products, the Pure Food and Drug Act of 1906. In 1912, Congress amended the Pure Food and Drug Act (the Sherley Amendment) to prohibit manufacturers from labeling drugs with false therapeutic claims that would mislead the purchaser.

Prior to 1930, the Food and Drug Administration (FDA) was known as the Food, Drug and Insecticide Administration. In 1930, the name was officially changed to the Food and Drug Administration. In 1933, FDA recommended a complete revision of the 1906 Pure Food and Drugs Act, leading to legislative efforts over the next 5 years to enact the legislative changes. The pivotal event leading to passage of the 1938 FDCA occurred in 1937 when more than 100 persons, including many children, died after taking a drug (sulfanilamide elixir) that had been marketed without adequate safety testing. Unfortunately, the drug contained a poisonous substance (diethylene glycol, the ingredient used in antifreeze) and the manufacturer did not conduct safety tests before selling the product.

The FDCA established many new requirements to ensure the safety, efficacy, and purity of drugs and other products (**Box 3-1**). The law extended FDA jurisdiction for safety, quality, and purity requirements to cosmetics and medical devices. The law required that drugs be proven safe for their intended uses before they are marketed and required inspections of manufacturing facilities. The law made it easier for the FDA to prove that a manufacturer intended to defraud consumers with false therapeutic claims for a misbranding violation. The FDCA has been amended a number of times since its initial passage in 1938 to add further protections for the safety and purity of drugs.

The FDCA drug approval process is well established. Some requirements include manufacturer applications to FDA, and FDA's monitoring and review of the

---

Box 3-1
Actions Resulting from the
Food, Drug, and Cosmetic Act of 1938

- Added FDA control over cosmetics and medical devices
- Required new drugs to be shown safe before marketing
- Removed the requirement to prove intent to deceive for misbranded drugs
- Authorized inspections of manufacturing facilities
- Allowed FDA to seek injunction remedy

---

drug and its testing process before approving a drug for use in the United States. This process is covered in Chapter 4.

A major amendment to the FDCA occurred in 1951 with the Durham–Humphrey Amendment (also known as the Prescription Drug Amendment). The Durham–Humphrey Amendment requires certain drugs to be dispensed only pursuant to a prescription, and requires that any refills be authorized either in the original prescription or by the prescriber. The basis of this amendment was FDA determination that certain drugs required medical supervision to be used safely. The amendment established the "legend" (i.e., prescription drug) requirement to distinguish prescription drugs from over-the-counter drugs by requiring that they be labeled with the following phrase:

> Caution: Federal law prohibits dispensing without a prescription.

The "legend" phrase has now been replaced with the requirement for prescription drugs to be labeled with the term "RxOnly." With the advent of prescription-only drugs, the amendment included an exemption to allow pharmacist labeling of patient prescription containers to meet the FDCA drug labeling requirement. The amendment also allows the FDA to switch prescription drugs to over-the-counter (OTC) status.

 Key Point

The Durham–Humphrey Amendment requires certain drugs to be dispensed only pursuant to a prescription, and required that any refills be authorized either in the original prescription or by the prescriber.

The FDCA was amended to add even stronger drug safety provisions after the sleeping medication thalidomide caused serious birth defects in thousands of children in Europe whose mothers had been given the drug during pregnancy.

The drug was not approved for use in the United States. In 1962, in response to the thalidomide tragedy, Congress enacted the Kefauver–Harris Amendments to the FDCA to require drug manufacturers to now show that the drug is *efficacious* and has greater drug safety for FDA approval. For the 4000 drugs approved between 1938 and 1962, FDA began efficacy studies in the late 1960s. Drugs on the market prior to the 1938 enactment of the FDCA were not subject to this review, although many have since been reviewed.

FDA has taken a role in the information that patients receive about their prescription drugs. For certain prescription drugs, FDA requires that pharmacists provide patients with a *patient package insert* or "PPI."[2] One of the earliest patient package inserts, for patients on oral contraceptives, became available in 1970.[3] PPIs are different from the manufacturer's drug product information for physicians and pharmacists (called the *package insert*). PPIs are for patient use to provide them with information about the risks and benefits and proper use of a prescription drug. On the other hand, the package insert is designed to provide physicians and pharmacists with more detailed information on prescription drugs such as the indications for use, recommended dose and route of administration, potential risks and adverse reactions, and other information necessary for proper use of the drug.

FDA has another program to provide patients with information about their prescribed drugs known as Medication Guides or Medguides. FDA requires Medguides for certain drugs that it determines have the potential to cause serious or significant side effects. More information on Medguides is available on FDA's website at http://www.fda.gov/cder/Offices/ODS/medication_guides.htm.

The Drug Listing Act of 1972 amended the Food, Drug, and Cosmetic Act to require drug manufacturers, repackagers, and companies that relabel drug products to register their facilities and provide a listing of all drugs they distribute commercially, including the drug's trade name and the drug's identifying number. That number is called the National Drug Code or NDC number. Pharmacies routinely use drug NDC numbers for many reasons, including identification of the dispensed drug. The NDC number contains three segments where each of the three numbers has a meaning. The first set of numbers identifies the drug manufacturer or company that labeled the product. The second set of numbers identifies the product strength and size, and the third set of numbers identifies the package size (e.g., 100).

The Orphan Drug Act of 1983 and its amendments encourage drug manufacturers to research and develop drugs to treat rare diseases affecting small numbers of U.S. residents. Because research and development of drugs to treat these rare diseases would be costly and the likelihood of profitability uncertain, the law gives drug companies incentives to research and develop these drugs (e.g., tax credits for clinical testing and specific years after FDA approval to exclusively market the drug). Examples of rare diseases include Lou Gehrig's disease, muscular dystrophy, and Huntington's disease. Since the law was enacted, more than 200 drug products have been approved as orphan drugs. One example of an orphan drug is Epogen® (erythropoietin).

In 1984, the Drug Price Competition and Patent Term Restoration Act (also called the Hatch–Waxman Act) was enacted. The law allows an accelerated process for FDA approval of generic drugs by not requiring generic drug manufacturers to repeat the research required for approval of the brand drug product. The law allows generic drug manufacturers applying for FDA approval to show that the generic drug is therapeutically equivalent to an already FDA-approved brand drug. The law also allows a drug manufacturer to apply for additional years of patent protection for its brand drug to recover time lost while the drug is awaiting FDA approval for marketing.

In 1988, the Prescription Drug Marketing Act of 1987 (PDMA) was signed into law. PDMA added protections to ensure the safety of prescription drugs by taking steps to prevent counterfeit, substandard, ineffective, or expired prescription drugs from entering the U.S. drug distribution system. Congress enacted PDMA to address problems from drug diversion and the risk of counterfeit drugs. PDMA added requirements for control over the wholesale drug distribution system, including state licensure of wholesale drug distributors. PDMA also requires unauthorized distributors of prescription drugs (i.e., not the manufacturers or the authorized wholesale distributors) to provide a statement (commonly known as a "pedigree") to the purchaser showing the prior sales history of the drug. PDMA also prohibited the resale of drugs purchased by hospitals or health care entities or donated to charitable organizations except in limited circumstances, restricted drug importation to only drug manufacturers, and prohibited the sale or purchase of drug samples.

In 1997, the Food and Drug Administration Modernization Act (FDAMA) was enacted. FDAMA established a number of changes to streamline and modernize FDA approval processes. The major change for pharmacists was to replace the legend statement "Caution: Federal law prohibits dispensing without a prescription" with the phrase "Rx Only" on the label of prescription drug products. Pharmacy technicians will be able to see the "RxOnly" labeling on the prescription drug products in the pharmacy. **Table 3-1** provides a timeline of major federal drug laws.

FDA's Enforcement Authority

FDA has authority to enforce the FDCA and other laws covering the quality and safety of prescription and over-the-counter drugs, medical devices, and other products such as animal drugs and food products. In the event of a problem with a drug product, FDA may work with the drug manufacturer to correct the problem

Table 3-1
Timeline of Federal Drug Laws

1906	Pure Food and Drug Act
1912	Sherley Amendment
1930	Food and Drug Administration named
1938	Congress passes the Food, Drug, and Cosmetic Act (FDCA) of 1938
1951	Durham–Humphrey Amendment to FDCA
1962	Kefauver–Harris Amendment to FDCA
1970	FDA requires the first patient package insert for oral contraceptives
1972	Drug Listing Act
1983	Orphan Drug Act
1984	Drug Price Competition and Patent Term Restoration Act
1988	Prescription Drug Marketing Act
1997	Food and Drug Administration Modernization Act

and may ask the manufacturer to voluntarily recall the product. FDA may take administrative enforcement actions, and also has the option of legal actions such as an injunction or fines or criminal penalties for intentional violations.

The FDCA establishes a number of prohibited acts, that is, actions that manufacturers and distributors may not engage in. Examples of prohibited acts include:

▶ Introducing any adulterated or misbranded drug, device, food, or cosmetic into the market.
▶ Making any adulterated or misbranded drug, device, food, or cosmetic.
▶ Receiving any adulterated or misbranded drug, device, food, or cosmetic.
▶ Manufacturing any adulterated or misbranded drug, device, food, or cosmetic.
▶ Selling or dispensing any counterfeit drug.
▶ Engaging in any acts that cause a drug to be counterfeit.

FDA has authority to request that a drug be recalled from the market due to quality or safety concerns. A drug recall may occur after a problem is reported to the FDA. Reports to FDA about potential problems with a particular drug may come from many sources, including pharmacists. FDA investigates and evaluates the reports and may request that a manufacturer recall a drug product. FDA classifies recalls into three categories, as shown in **Table 3-2**.

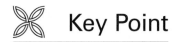 **Key Point**

FDA has authority to request or order that a drug be recalled from the market due to quality or safety concerns.

Table 3-2
FDA Drug Product Recalls

Class I	Dangerous or defective drug that could cause serious health problems
Class II	Drug that may cause a temporary health problem or threat of a serious problem
Class III	Drug is unlikely to cause a health problem, but may violate FDA labeling or manufacturing regulations

Drug recalls may involve recalling certain "batches" of a drug product or recalling all of a drug product. If a serious safety concern exists, FDA may request that a drug be *withdrawn* from the market that in practical terms generally leads to a permanent recall. This would occur if the FDA determines that the risks of the drug are serious and outweigh the benefits of leaving the drug on the market available for physicians to prescribe. An example occurred in 1997 when certain weight loss drugs were withdrawn after they were linked to serious health problems.

An important distinction relative to pharmacy is that regulation of the pharmacy profession is handled by the states. However, federal regulation of drug distribution and manufacturing has indirect effects on the practice of pharmacy. For instance, FDA has authority over the quality and efficacy of drugs that are dispensed by pharmacists, and FDA considers drugs dispensed within the United States without a valid prescription to be "misbranded" under the FDCA. In addition, the requirements in the Omnibus Budget Reconciliation Act of 1990 (discussed later in this chapter) indirectly affect pharmacy practice by requiring patient counseling, drug use review, and records for Medicaid patients.

 Key Point

If a serious safety concern exists, FDA may request that a drug be *withdrawn* from the market which, in practical terms, leads to a permanent recall.

Poison Prevention Packaging Act

In 1970, Congress enacted the Poison Prevention Packaging Act.[4] The Consumer Product Safety Commission (CPSC) is the federal agency responsible for enforcing the law. The law requires that hazardous products such as household cleaners, furniture polish, prescription drugs, and over-the-counter drug products be sold in *child-resistant* packaging that will prevent children from opening the package but allow adults to open the containers without difficulty. The law requires that child-resistant packaging undergo specific testing with children under 5 years of age and separately with adults. The first test on children must show that at least 85% of the children are unable to open the packaging in a 5-minute period. For the second part of the test, children that are unable to open the packaging are shown how to open the packaging and given another 5 minutes to open the package. At least 80% of the children must be unable to open the packaging in the second test. For the adult-testing phase, at least 90% of tested adults should be able to open and close the packaging with relative ease.

There are exceptions to the child-resistant packaging requirement. Consumers may ask the pharmacist to dispense their prescription in non-child-resistant packaging. On prescriptions, medical practitioners may ask for non-child-resistant packaging for their patients. In such instances, pharmacists are permitted to dispense the drugs in non-child resistant containers. In addition, some prescription drugs are exempt from child-resistant packaging because it is not appropriate, feasible, or practical. For example, sublingual nitroglycerin tablets are not in child-resistant packaging so that patients may have quick access to the medication. The CPSC is allowed to exempt certain products if child-resistant packaging is not needed to protect children. Examples of medications not packaged in child-resistant packaging include oral contraceptives in cyclical packaging. The following is a list of drugs that are exempt from child-resistant packaging:

▶ Bulk prescription drug products intended for repackaging by pharmacists in dispensing prescription drugs
▶ Prescription drugs dispensed in institutional facilities such as hospitals and nursing homes
▶ Sublingual nitroglycerin
▶ Sublingual and chewable isosorbide dinitrate (Isordil®)
▶ Oral contraceptives in the manufacturers' dispenser packages
▶ Cholestyramine powder packets
▶ Corticosteroid tablets in manufacturer dispensing packages
▶ Topical ointments and creams

Many over-the-counter drugs require child-resistant packaging. Examples include products containing aspirin, acetaminophen, ibuprofen, iron, and fluoride. OTC products that are packaged in non-child-resistant packaging must be labeled clearly to warn against having these products in households with young children. The required statement is: "This Package Is for Households without Young Children."

Omnibus Budget Reconciliation Act of 1990 (OBRA '90)

In 1990, Congress enacted the Omnibus Budget Reconciliation Act of 1990 (commonly known as OBRA '90). OBRA '90 has requirements for pharmacists that dispense medications for state Medicaid patients. These requirements include pharmacist-provided drug use review (DUR), patient counseling, and specific patient records. Drug use review (DUR) requires pharmacists to review a patient's drug treatment for any drug therapy problems such as drug interactions, incorrect drug dosage, and potential for drug misuse or abuse.

OBRA '90 also required states to issue rules for pharmacist patient counseling. Pharmacists are required to offer counseling to patients on matters such as how to take the drug, how long to take the drug, common side effects, how to avoid contraindications, drugs or foods that should not be taken with the drug, proper drug storage, what to do if a dose is missed, and information on refilling their medication.

For patient records, OBRA '90 requires pharmacists to make reasonable efforts to keep certain information on Medicaid patients such as patient name, address, telephone number, age, sex, and individual history including disease states, known allergies, drug reactions, a list of medications, and any comments from the pharmacist about the patient's drug therapy.

Medicare Modernization Act of 2003

Medicare was enacted in 1965 to provide health care insurance benefits to the United State's senior population and to disabled persons. When Medicare was enacted, it did not pay for outpatient prescription drugs. The law primarily covered drugs provided to Medicare patients while hospitalized and drugs that patients could not self-administer. Medicare did not pay for outpatient prescription drugs. A possible reason for not covering outpatient drugs is that prescription drugs played a lesser role in health care treatment at that time. However, the role of prescription drug therapy has changed dramatically.

 Key Point

When Medicare was first enacted, it did not pay for outpatient prescription drugs.

Prescription drugs now have a major role in treating many diseases such as high blood pressure, high cholesterol, diabetes, infectious diseases, and many other conditions. Adding coverage for outpatient prescription drugs to Medicare has been a goal for many years. In 2003, one of the most significant changes to federal laws affecting pharmacy occurred. The Medicare Prescription Drug, Improvement, and Modernization Act of 2003 added an outpatient prescription drug benefit to Medicare. The new Medicare law also offers patients who take many prescription drugs and have numerous chronic diseases the right to have their medication therapy reviewed by pharmacists and other health care providers. The service is called medication therapy management (MTM). Although the law does not require that MTM be provided by pharmacists, they are well suited to provide MTM with their extensive education and training on drug therapy.

 Key Point

The Medicare Prescription Drug, Improvement, and Modernization Act of 2003 added a prescription drug benefit to Medicare.

Summary

Prescription drugs are covered by numerous federal laws and regulations. The Food, Drug, and Cosmetic Act is the primary federal law establishing requirements for drugs available in the United States to ensure that they are safe, effective, and accompanied by proper information and warnings for their use. The efforts to enact U.S. drug laws to control the safety and quality of drugs and to protect the public from unsafe and poorly labeled drugs began in the 1800s. The first drug safety law, the Pure Food and Drug Act, was enacted in 1906 followed in 1938 by enactment of the federal Food, Drug, and Cosmetic Act (FDCA). The FDCA sets requirements to provide for safety, efficacy, quality, and purity of drugs and other products. The FDCA has been amended many times since being enacted, including a 1951 amendment to require certain drugs to be dispensed only by prescription.

The Food and Drug Administration (FDA) is the federal agency with authority over drug manufacturers and enforcement of the FDCA. FDA regulates many areas related to drugs such as the labeling of prescription drugs and over-the-counter drugs, certain information that patients receive about their prescription drugs, protections to prevent counterfeit and adulterated drugs from entering the drug supply, and recalls of drugs due to safety concerns. Other federal laws applicable to drugs that affect the practice of pharmacy include the Poison Prevention Packaging Act requiring the use of child-resistant packaging, the Omnibus Budget Reconciliation Act of 1990 setting requirements for counseling patients on their prescribed medications, and the Medicare law of 2003 providing coverage for outpatient prescription drugs for Medicare beneficiaries.

References

1. 21 U.S. Code Sections 301 *et. seq.*
2. See the Internet link to the FDA Office of Drug Safety at http://www.fda.gov/cder/Offices/ODS/labeling.htm.
3. 21 CFR section 310.510.
4. 15 U.S.C. 1471 *et. seq*

Self-Assessment Questions

1. The FDCA includes comprehensive requirements for what areas of drug distribution in the United States?
2. The PPI (patient package insert) provides drug information for patients or consumers, while the package insert is intended for whom?
3. What was the significance of the Durham–Humphrey Amendment to the FDCA?
4. What government agency enforces the FDCA?
5. What is meant by MTM?

Chapter 4

Food and Drug Administration

Chapter Outline

Learning Objectives

1. Identify the FDA centers and their roles.
2. Describe the drug approval process.
3. Define brand name drug.
4. Compare and contrast brand name drugs and therapeutically equivalent generic drugs.
5. Define therapeutically equivalent generic drug.
6. Discuss information found in the "Orange Book."
7. Compare and contrast the labels on a finished drug product package and an over-the-counter drug.
8. Define the expiration date and beyond-use date of a medication.
9. Discuss the use of and need for a lot number.

Introduction

The goal of this chapter is to provide an overview of the organization of the Food and Drug Administration (FDA) and the FDA's role in assuring the safety and efficacy of drugs in the United States. This chapter outlines the FDA's policies and regulatory responsibilities, the drug approval process, therapeutically equivalent drugs, labeling for prescription and over-the-counter drug products, the use of expiration dates, and beyond-use dating.

The Organization

The Food and Drug Administration (FDA) is responsible for protecting public health by assuring the safety and efficacy of a number of products available in the United States, including human drugs, veterinary drugs, medical devices, food, cosmetics, and biological products. FDA's mission statement (**Box 4-1**) details its role in protecting public health. FDA regulates a large number of companies engaged in manufacturing and distributing these products.

FDA is a federal agency within the Department of Health and Human Services. FDA is one of the largest federal agencies. It is organized into eight different units consisting of five centers, the Office of the FDA Commissioner, the Office of Regulatory Affairs, and the National Center for Toxicological Research. The five centers provide regulatory oversight of different categories of products (**Box 4-2**).

The Office of the Commissioner is comprised of several other offices such as the Office of Policy and Planning, Office of Legislation, and Office of the Chief Counsel. The Office of Regulatory Affairs assists the Commissioner with compliance, enforcement, and regulation of facilities that manufacture the products under FDA regulatory authority. The Office's agents inspect these facilities to assure that the products meet the FDA standards for manufacturing, labeling, and

---

Box 4-1
FDA's Mission Statement

The FDA is responsible for protecting the public health by assuring the safety, efficacy, and security of human and veterinary drugs, biological products, medical devices, our nation's food supply, cosmetics, and products that emit radiation. The FDA is also responsible for advancing the public health by helping to speed innovations that make medicines and foods more effective, safer, and more affordable; and helping the public get the accurate, science-based information they need to use medicines and foods to improve their health.

http://www.fda.gov/opacom/morechoices/mission.html

> ## Box 4-2
> ## FDA Centers
>
> - The Center for Biologics Evaluation and Research (CBER)—responsible for safety of blood products, allergen tests and treatments, vaccines, and new therapeutic products from stem cells and gene therapy.
> - The Center for Devices and Radiologic Health (CDRH)—responsible for reviewing and regulating medical devices and radiation products such as x-rays.
> - The Center for Drug Evaluation and Research (CDER)—responsible for reviewing and assuring the safety of new drugs, generic drugs, and over-the-counter drugs.
> - The Center for Food Safety and Applied Nutrition (CFSAN)—responsible for safety of cosmetics, food, seafood, food additives, color additives, food packaging, dairy products, dietary supplements, and infant formula.
> - The Center for Veterinary Medicine (CVM)—responsible for animal drugs, animal feed, and feed ingredients.

other requirements. The National Center for Toxicological Research assists with scientific research needed by the FDA.

FDA does not directly regulate pharmacy practice because the states regulate the practice of pharmacy. However, there are areas where FDA actions affect the practice of pharmacy. For example, for some drugs, FDA requires pharmacies to provide patients with a patient package insert with dispensed prescriptions. In addition, FDA regulates drug manufacturing, and in some instances FDA has expressed concerns that pharmacy drug compounding is similar to drug manufacturing.

Pharmacists have a long-standing practice of drug compounding. The Food, Drug, and Cosmetic Act of 1938 (FDCA) exempts pharmacies from registering as drug manufacturers if they prepare and dispense drugs, including drug compounding, in the regular course of business as a retail pharmacy.[1] FDA relies on the state Boards of Pharmacy to regulate pharmacies engaged in drug compounding. However, FDA has advised that it would consider enforcement actions against pharmacies if it finds that a pharmacy's drug compounding activities amounted to drug manufacturing subject to regulation under the FDCA.

Federal Approval of Drugs

FDA approves drugs that are available for distribution and marketing in the United States, including prescription and over-the-counter drugs (**Table 4-1**). FDA will not approve drugs for distribution and marketing in the United States until the drugs are shown to be safe and effective.

When a drug company discovers a new drug, the company submits a new drug application (known as an NDA) to FDA to obtain approval for distribution and

Table 4-1
FDA Drug Approval Process

Preclinical Research
Drug development and animal tests
↓

Investigational New Drug Application
Filed with the FDA
↓

Clinical Trials (Studies)
- Phase I
- Phase II
- Phase III
↓

New Drug Application (NDA)
Filed with the FDA
↓

FDA Review and Approval
The FDA may take up to 2 years or longer before issuing its decision on approval of the drug
↓

Post-Marketing Surveillance
Monitor ongoing safety after FDA has approved the drug for marketing and distribution

marketing of the drug in the United States. FDA review of a new drug for approval includes consideration of the benefits of the drug, the potential risks with using the drug, and other factors. The time from the initial development of the drug until the drug receives final FDA approval may take a number of years, up to 10 years or longer in some instances. However, FDA has the option to give an accelerated approval process to new drugs that show promise in treating serious or life-threatening diseases.

 Key Point

FDA will not approve drugs for distribution and marketing in the United States until the drugs are shown to be safe and effective.

Drugs begin their development process when they are discovered through research by a drug manufacturer. If the drug manufacturer continues development of the drug, the following are the general steps to evaluate the drug's safety and effectiveness:

▶ Preclinical research
▶ Filing an investigational new drug (IND) application

- ❯ Clinical trials (studies) consisting of Phase I, II, and III
- ❯ Filing a new drug application (NDA)
- ❯ FDA review and approval process
- ❯ Final FDA approval of the drug

Preclinical research involves a drug manufacturer 1) searching for new drug compounds that have the potential to be used as treatment for certain diseases or conditions and 2) conducting animal tests and initial safety testing. If the drug is promising, the drug manufacturer files an investigational new drug (IND) application with FDA. If the IND is approved by FDA, the drug manufacturer is permitted to start the investigational clinical trials with the drug in humans. The human clinical testing is done in three phases: Phase I, II, and III. Phase I evaluates the drug's proper safe dosage. Phase II evaluates the drug's effectiveness, side effects, and risks. Phase III clinical studies continue the safety and effectiveness testing. Next, if the drug has so far been shown to be safe and effective, the drug manufacturer files a new drug application (NDA). The NDA contains all of the drug's scientific and clinical study information. If FDA approves the NDA and issues a final approval letter, the new drug is approved for use. However, before the drug may be marketed and distributed, FDA must also approve the drug's product labeling, including the package insert. FDA continues to monitor approved drugs for safety and effectiveness after approval through post-marketing surveillance programs. If unacceptable adverse risks occur, FDA has options such as requiring that the drug manufacturer change the product's package insert to add particular warnings.

Brand Name Drugs and Generic Drugs

A brand name drug is an FDA-approved drug that is marketed under the drug manufacturer's trade name (also known as the brand name). Lipitor® is an example of a brand or trade name for a drug that is manufactured and distributed by Pfizer, the drug's manufacturer. The generic name for the drug in Lipitor® is lovastatin. Another example of a generic drug name is ibuprofen, which is the drug contained in the brand name drugs Advil® and Motrin®.

Drug manufacturers obtain patents for new drugs they develop. During the term of the patent, only the drug company that holds the patent is allowed to market and distribute the drug. After the patent expires, other drug companies may seek approval from the FDA to manufacture the same drug with the identical active drug as the brand name drug. These are known as the generically equivalent drugs (i.e., they are generically equivalent to the brand name drug). Although the patent has expired, the original drug manufacturer retains the sole right to use the brand name for the drug.

The generic drug is the same as the brand name drug. It has the same dosage form (e.g., capsule), strength (e.g., number of grams or milligrams), route of administration (e.g., oral), and treatment indications. Generic drugs must be approved by FDA for use and distribution in the United States. Generic drugs are required to meet the same FDA standards for manufacturing and quality as brand drugs. Generic drugs look different than the brand name drug because the laws do not allow a generic drug to copy the appearance of the brand name drug. However, a generic drug contains the same active ingredient. Generic drug companies distribute the drug under the generic name.

Before a generic drug company is permitted to market and distribute a generically equivalent drug, the drug manufacturer must establish to FDA that its generic drug is therapeutically equivalent to the brand drug. The generic drug company must show that the generic drug has the same active ingredient, strength, dosage form (e.g., tablet or liquid), and bioequivalence (meaning that the generic drug's active ingredient is absorbed at the same rate and extent as the brand drug). The generic drug company must also show that the drug meets the FDA manufacturing and quality control requirements and that the drug will retain its potency until the expiration date.

Generic Drug Substitution

Every state has laws and regulations establishing the requirements that pharmacists are required to follow when they engage in substituting a generic drug for a brand name drug. These are called generic substitution laws and regulations. State generic substitution laws and regulations allow pharmacists to substitute therapeutically equivalent generic drugs for prescribed brand name drugs unless the prescriber requests that generic substitution not occur. The prescriber may request no substitution for the prescribed drug either with the prescription or through oral instructions to the pharmacist. Patients may also ask to have the brand name drug dispensed rather than the generic drug. In some states, pharmacists are required to do generic substitution for certain types of patients such as patients with prescription drug coverage paid for by the state medical assistance program.

 Key Point

Every state has laws and regulations establishing the requirements that pharmacists are required to follow when they engage in "generic substitution."

State laws establish different means for prescribers to advise pharmacists to dispense the brand name drug (i.e., not substitute the generic drug for their patients). Depending on the state, the laws may instruct prescribers to indicate no substitution through various phrases on the prescription, including "dispense as written," "DAW," "no substitution," "do not substitute," or words of similar effect. Conversely, if the prescriber wants to permit substitution, state laws may instruct the prescriber to use terms such as "substitution permitted" or words of similar effect. Some state laws require that specific terms be used to prevent generic substitution, and some states require prescription blanks to have special boxes to check or require the prescriber to sign on a particular line to prevent generic substitution.

FDA provides a list of generic drugs that the agency has found to be therapeutically equivalent for generic substitution for the brand name drugs in its publication called the *Approved Drug Products with Therapeutic Equivalence Evaluations* (commonly called the "Orange Book"). Pharmacists use the "Orange Book" to find FDA's determination that a particular manufacturer's generic drug is therapeutically equivalent to the brand name drug.

The "Orange Book" uses a set of codes to indicate the therapeutic equivalency of the generic drugs in comparison to the brand name drugs (**Table 4-2**). For example, oral capsules and tablets of generic drugs that have been determined by the FDA to be therapeutically equivalent to the brand name drug are rated "AA" or "AB." If drugs are rated therapeutically equivalent, then the generic drug may be substituted for the brand name drug with the assurance that the same therapeutic effect will occur. The FDA "Orange Book" also has codes for drugs that have been found by FDA to *not* be therapeutically equivalent.

Table 4-2
"Orange Book" Codes for Therapeutic Equivalence for Oral Drugs

FDA Codes for Therapeutic Equivalence for Oral Drugs	FDA Codes
Drug products that FDA considers to be therapeutically equivalent to other pharmaceutically equivalent products having no known or suspected bioequivalence problems.	AA, AN, AO, AP, or AT, depending on the dosage form
Drug products for which actual or potential bioequivalence problems have been resolved with adequate in vivo or in vitro evidence supporting the bioequivalence.	AB
Drug products that the FDA considers *not* to be therapeutically equivalent to other pharmaceutically equivalent products (i.e., drug products for which actual or potential bioequivalence problems have not been resolved by adequate evidence of bioequivalence).	BC, BD, BE, BN, BP, BR, BS, BT, BX, or B

Prescription Drug Labeling and Package Inserts

In addition to the safety and effectiveness of drugs, FDA regulates drug product labeling. Prescription drug products are packaged in finished drug product packages (e.g., bottles, tubes) that are prepared and labeled by the drug manufacturer. The information that drug manufacturers are required to put on the finished drug container label is regulated by the FDCA and federal drug labeling regulations.[2] The requirements for the container label include a number of items such as the name and address of the manufacturer, packager, or distributor; drug brand name and generic name; expiration date; active ingredient(s) and amount per dosage form; quantity; usual recommended dose or reference to package insert; "Rx Only" to indicate prescription only; route of administration; lot number or control number; and information on the proper storage and temperature requirements.

Federal regulations require drug manufacturers to provide prescribing and other additional information with prescription drugs. This information is contained in the package insert. The package insert provides physicians, pharmacists, and other health care professionals with the medical and scientific information about the prescription drug. FDA regulations require the package insert to contain the following information:

▶ A summary of the scientific information for the safe and effective use of the drug.

▶ Specific sections covering information described below.

   ◆ *Description*: includes the proprietary and established name of the drug, the dosage form (e.g., tablet, capsule, cream), route of administration (e.g., oral, topical, injection), ingredients, therapeutic or pharmacologic class of the drug (e.g., antibiotic, anti-hypertensive for high blood pressure), the chemical name and structure of the drug, and other information about the drug.

   ◆ *Clinical Pharmacology*: includes information on how the drug acts on the human body to produce its beneficial effect, and other information such as how it is absorbed and how long its therapeutic levels last.

   ◆ *Indication and Usage*: provides information on the diseases and conditions for which the drug is indicated (e.g., ampicillin is indicated for the treatment of infections caused by susceptible bacteria, or the drug is indicated to treat a condition such as hypertension for high blood pressure) and other information such as how to monitor patients while taking the medication.

   ◆ *Contraindications*: provides information on situations where the drug should not be used (i.e., its use is contraindicated because the risks from using the drug are greater than the benefits of therapy).

- ◆ *Warnings*: describes serious adverse reactions and potential safety concerns, and is revised quickly if a new potential risk is believed to be associated with a drug. For special risks that are very serious and may result in death or serious injury, the FDA may require that a special warning be put in the package insert (commonly called a *"black box warning"* because the warning is usually emphasized inside a box).

- ◆ *Precautions*: contains information on precautions that should be considered for the safe and effective use of the drug, such as *information for patients;* laboratory tests to assist with monitoring the drug's use; potential interactions between the drug and other drugs or laboratory tests; use in pregnant patients, nursing mothers, children, and elderly patients; and other precautions to consider.

- ◆ *Adverse Reactions*: are undesirable effects that may occur when a drug is used. This section provides a list of the adverse reactions that have been associated with or may occur with the drug's use.

- ◆ *Drug Abuse and Dependence*: provides information on the drug's potential for abuse and dependence, if any.

- ◆ *Overdosage*: discusses the signs and symptoms that occur with an overdose of the drug.

- ◆ *Dosage and Administration*: addresses the proper dosage and administration of the drug for safe and effective use, including the recommended and usual dosages, the frequency of administration (e.g., number of doses per day), and the duration of treatment.

- ◆ *How Supplied*: covers the dosage form and strength for the drug (e.g., 100 mg capsules, 50 mg tablets, or liquid with 5 mg/5 ml).

- ◆ *Animal Pharmacology and Animal Toxicology*: is not always included. It provides information on any animal testing and results.

- ◆ *Clinical Studies and References*: provides information on clinical studies on the drug's use and effect that have been done in humans.

In 2006, FDA revised the package insert requirements.[3] The goal of the package insert changes was to highlight important drug information on prescription drugs, and focus attention on the most important information. These changes apply to new and recently approved prescription drug products. Some of the changes include a highlights section with information that health care professionals commonly use, a separate patient counseling section to emphasize communications between the patient and health care professionals, and a telephone number for reporting suspected side effects. These revisions are intended to make it easier for pharmacists, physicians, and other health care professionals to read and use the package insert information, and aid the safe and effective use of prescription drug products.

Over-the-Counter Drug Labeling

FDA also sets requirements for labeling of over-the-counter (OTC or nonprescription) drugs. The major difference between the labeling for prescription drugs and OTC drugs is that the OTC labeling is designed for use by the consumer. OTC drug products are labeled with the drug's brand name or generic drug name and strength and the total quantity of drugs in the container. This labeling is intended to sufficiently inform the consumer of the indication for the drug, the recommended dosage, how often the drug may be taken, and who should or should not take the medication. The labeling also provides information on the potential side effects and precautions for using the drug. For instance, the container labeling for OTC drugs used for sleep aids would advise the consumer not to drive a car after taking the medication due to the risk of drowsiness.

 Key Point

The major difference between the labeling for prescription drugs and OTC drugs is that the OTC labeling is designed for use by the consumer.

New FDA rules for the labeling of OTC products became effective in 2002 for some products and for all products in 2005.[4] Under the new rules, FDA requires OTC drugs to be labeled with a *Drug Facts* label that contains the following sections:

- *Active Ingredient*: provides the active ingredient and its amount in each dosage unit (e.g., ibuprofen 200 mg in each capsule). It also provides the purposes for the medication use (e.g., pain reliever).
- *Uses*: provides the recommended uses for the drug.
- *Warnings*: provides warnings on adverse effects that could potentially occur with the use of the medication, allergy alerts, risks of using the drug if it is taken with other products such as drugs or alcohol, and when the medication should not be taken (e.g., if the patient is allergic to the medication or pregnant or has some other conditions).
- *Directions*: gives the consumer information on the recommended dose and frequency for taking the drug, maximum dosage, and information on using the drug in children.
- *Other Information:* provides other information on safe storage of the drug such as temperature and humidity.

The new OTC labeling requirements mandate standardized content and format to make OTC product information easier to understand for consumers.

Pharmacy technicians may be asked questions about the use of OTC drugs. You should refer questions to the pharmacist.

Expiration Dates, Beyond-Use Dates, and Lot Numbers

Drug manufacturers are required by FDA to label their drug products with an expiration date.[5] The expiration date is based on the stability of the drug in the manufacturer's original container and is the date after which the drug manufacturer no longer guarantees the full potency and safety of the drug product. The expiration date is determined by studies conducted by the drug manufacturer.[6] The date is used to determine how long the drug product may be used or dispensed to patients. Drugs that have reached their expiration date may not be used or dispensed to patients. It is important to check the expiration date on the manufacturer's container *each* time a drug is dispensed or used.

 Key Point

The expiration date on the drug's original container is derived from studies conducted by the drug manufacturer on the stability of the drug in the manufacturer's container.[7]

Pharmacists place a "beyond-use" date on the prescription container label. The United States Pharmacopoeia (USP) defines the beyond-use date as the date after which the drug should be discarded and no longer used by the patient. State pharmacy laws and regulations require pharmacists to place a beyond-use date on the labeling of the prescription container and other pharmacy prepared drug products. For most oral dispensed drugs, the beyond-use date is usually the earlier of the manufacturer's expiration date or 1 year from the date that the drug is dispensed. For single-unit and unit dose containers, the date is a maximum of 1 year unless the manufacturer's labeling recommends a shorter date.

The beyond-use date is earlier for a number of reasons, including the opening of the manufacturer's original package, dispensing or repackaging the drug into a different container than the manufacturer's original container, different storage conditions after the drug is dispensed, storage in a patient's home, and frequent opening of the prescription container after dispensing. Exceptions to the beyond-use date exist for certain drugs. For example, some medications that are reconstituted before use or dispensing have special shorter beyond-use dates after reconstitution (usually in terms of days). The manufacturer's labeling will provide information on these special beyond-use dates. Pharmacies do not reconstitute oral powders such as oral antibiotic powders until the patient picks the medication up from the pharmacy, due to the shorter dating for reconstituted products, to ensure that the product is good for the length of time that the patient needs it.

FDA requires that the manufacturer's product container include a lot number or control number on the label. Federal regulations define the lot number (or control number) as a unique combination of letters, numbers, or symbols that may be used to find the complete history of the manufacturing and distribution of a batch or lot of a drug product.[8] The lot or control number is an important part of the information on the drug container label. From time to time, circumstances may occur where a particular lot of a drug product needs to be recalled from pharmacies and returned to the manufacturer. In the event of such a recall, the drug would usually be identified by the drug name and lot number and pharmacies would remove the recalled drugs from the pharmacy stock.

Summary

The Food and Drug Administration (FDA) is the federal agency with regulatory oversight and enforcement of laws governing the quality, safety, and efficacy of human and veterinary drugs, biological products, and other products, including medical devices, food, and cosmetics. FDA has a number of centers that cover the different FDA-regulated products such as the Center for Drug Evaluation and Research applicable to drugs. FDA approves drugs that are available for use in the United States by using a comprehensive approval process from initial drug discovery through clinical trials, final approval for distribution, and post-marketing surveillance after approval.

FDA reviews generic drug products to determine if they are therapeutically equivalent to the brand name drug product. Information on the FDA determination of therapeutically equivalent drug product approvals is provided in FDA's *Approved Drug Products with Therapeutic Equivalence Evaluations*, which is commonly called the "Orange Book." State laws and regulations establish requirements for pharmacists and prescribers to follow when an approved therapeutically equivalent generic drug is substituted for a brand name drug. FDA regulates the packaging and labeling for drug products with specific requirements for information that must be provided with prescription and over-the-counter drug products, including package labeling. In addition, FDA requires that drug products be labeled with expiration dates and a lot number.

References

1. See 21 U.S.C. Section 360(g).
2. Federal Food, Drug, and Cosmetic Act (21 U.S.C. § 301 et seq.) and 21 Code of Federal Regulations Part 201.
3. See FDA information at http://www.fda.gov/cder/regulatory/physLabel/summary.htm.
4. See 21 CFR 201.66.
5. See 21 CFR 211.137.
6. See 21 CFR 211.166.
7. See 21 CFR 211.166.
8. See 21 CFR 211.130.

Self-Assessment Questions

1. What is the FDA's role in protecting public health related to drug manufacturing and distribution in the United States?
2. What is a "generic drug?"
3. What do the generic substitution laws and regulations allow pharmacists to do when filling a prescription?
4. Non-prescription or OTC drug labeling is designed specifically for whom?
5. Drug expiration dates are derived from what type of drug studies?

Chapter 5

Controlled Substances Laws

Chapter Outline

Learning Objectives

1. List the five schedules of controlled substances and examples for each schedule.
2. Compare the five schedules based on risks for abuse, misuse, and dependency.
3. Identify requirements for controlled substance prescriptions, including information required from the physician and the pharmacy.
4. Describe the formula for determining the validity of a DEA number.
5. List the federal Controlled Substances Act requirements for the prescription label that is placed on a patient's container.
6. List the different DEA forms and their uses.

Introduction

Controlled substances are subject to more stringent controls by federal and state laws (and the implementing regulations) than other drugs because of the potential for misuse, abuse, diversion, and addiction. Controlled substances are used to treat a number of medical conditions such as pain, anxiety, seizures, and insomnia. Controlled substances laws and regulations establish a number of requirements for ordering, distribution, storage, recordkeeping, and handling of controlled substances by pharmacists as well as drug manufacturers, drug distributors, physicians, and other health care providers.

This chapter focuses on the *federal* controlled substances laws and regulations including schedules of controlled substances, labeling of controlled substances, prescribing and dispensing of controlled substances, transferring of controlled substance prescriptions, the Drug Enforcement Administration, ordering of controlled substances, and reporting of thefts and losses of controlled substances. The chapter also discusses state prescription monitoring programs and federal and state restrictions over the sales of products containing ephedrine, pseudoephedrine, and phenylpropanoloamine. State controlled substances laws and regulations vary from state to state and coverage. Decisions regarding dispensing of controlled substances prescriptions rest with the pharmacist. Pharmacists have responsibilities under controlled substances laws to dispense valid controlled substance prescriptions issued for a legitimate medical purpose. The Drug Enforcement Administration (DEA) Pharmacists' Manual available from the DEA provides information to assist pharmacists' understanding of the federal controlled substances laws. See http://www.deadiversion.usdoj.gov/pubs/manuals/index.html. Controlled substances laws and regulations are subject to change, and pharmacy technicians should defer to the pharmacist regarding dispensing of controlled substances.

 Key Point

Controlled substances are subject to more stringent controls by federal and state laws (and the implementing regulations) than other drugs because of the potential for misuse, abuse, diversion, and addiction.

Controlled Substances Laws

State and federal controlled substance laws add another layer of controls over drugs classified as controlled substances or regulated chemicals that apply to the practice of pharmacy. The federal Controlled Substances Act of 1970 or CSA,[1] and its regulations (21 Code of Federal Regulations Part 1300) establish comprehensive requirements and controls over the manufacture, import, export, distribution, ordering, dispensing, and prescribing of controlled substances and regulated chemicals. The Drug Enforcement Administration (DEA) is the primary federal agency enforcing the CSA. Under the CSA, the definition of controlled substances includes drugs and other substances and their immediate precursors. A precursor is a substance that may be turned into a controlled substance through a chemical reaction. Alcoholic beverages, including wine and beer, and also tobacco are not considered controlled substances.

States also have controlled substance laws and regulations. The federal laws and regulations set the minimum requirements. Therefore, state controlled substance laws and regulations may not be less strict than the federal controlled substance requirements, but may have additional stricter controls. Pharmacies must comply with the state laws for the jurisdiction where the pharmacy is located. If the state controlled substance law or regulation is stricter than the federal law or regulation, the stricter state requirements must be followed in addition to the federal law.

 ## Key Point

The stricter state controlled substances requirements must be followed in addition to the federal controlled substances requirements.

The federal Controlled Substances Act established a closed distribution system to tightly regulate the distribution and handling of controlled substances. The controls cover the distribution of controlled substances from the manufacture through the distribution, dispensing, storage, recordkeeping, and other actions involved with the distribution of controlled substances. An important aspect of these controls is the requirement to be registered with the DEA, including pharmacies, prescribers, drug manufacturers, and drug wholesale distributors in order to dispense or distribute controlled substances. Other controls include special forms for ordering controlled substances and reporting thefts or losses; maintaining inventories; keeping records of transactions; securing storage and transport of controlled substances; establishing controls over prescribing and dispensing; and instituting penalties against those who violate the controlled substance laws. These controls create a closed system to monitor the distribution and guard against abuse, misuse, and diversion of controlled substances throughout their handling and distribution process.

Schedules of Controlled Substances

The CSA established five schedules (classifications) for controlled substances: I, II, III, IV, and V. The CSA uses criteria (such as potential for abuse or addiction, medical use in the United States, scientific studies, and medical information on the drug's medical value) to determine the appropriate schedule for a controlled substance.[3] The schedule that a drug or substance is assigned determines its level of control. Schedule I is the most restrictive schedule, with Schedule V being the least controlled category of controlled substances.[4] Schedule I controlled substances are considered to have no accepted medical use, the highest potential for abuse, and are not available for prescribing, dispensing, or administration. Examples of Schedule I drugs include heroin and marijuana. Schedule II controlled substances have a high potential for abuse or misuse and psychological or physical dependence. Examples of Schedule II drugs include morphine, methadone, and codeine (not combined with other non-controlled drugs). Controlled substances in Schedules III, IV, and V have descending lesser potential risk of abuse and misuse. Schedule III drugs have some potential for abuse and risk of dependence that is less than Schedule II drugs but more than Schedule IV drugs. Examples of Schedule III drugs include Vicodin® and codeine combined with acetaminophen (Tylenol and Codeine®). Schedule IV drugs have a lower potential for abuse than Schedule III drugs but more potential than Schedule V drugs, and may cause limited dependence. Examples include Valium®, Ativan®, and Halcion®. Schedule V drugs have an abuse potential less than Schedule IV and primarily include products containing limited amounts of narcotic drugs used to treat cough or diarrhea.

Federal regulations classify some drug preparations as Schedule V.[5] Examples include cough medications with codeine such as Robitussin AC® and Phenergan with Codeine®, and preparations used to treat diarrhea such as Parepectolin (containing a small amount of opium) as well as products containing diphenoxylate with atropine (Lomotil®). The U.S. Drug Enforcement Administration maintains a website listing drugs and substances in the various schedules at http://www.usdoj.gov/dea/pubs/scheduling.html (**Table 5-1**).

Federal regulations allow certain controlled substances to be dispensed by a pharmacist (not by a nonpharmacist) without a prescription if specific requirements are met. These requirements include that the substance is not a prescription drug under the Food, Drug, and Cosmetic Act or any other federal, state, or local law, and the controlled substance is dispensed by a pharmacist.[6] Other requirements include pharmacist approval of the sale, the purchaser is at least 18 years of age, and a bound record book with information on the sale in the pharmacy. Information is maintained by the pharmacy that includes the purchaser's name and address, the name and quantity of the product purchased, the date of purchase, and the name or initials of the dispensing pharmacist. Once the pharmacist has met the requirements, the actual cash or credit sale may be completed by a nonpharmacist.

State laws vary on whether these Schedule V products may be sold without a prescription. Some states allow such CV products to be sold without a prescription, whereas other states restrict certain CV products (such as codeine cough preparations) to prescription only. State laws may have additional requirements beyond

Table 5-1
Schedules of Controlled Substances

Schedule	Classification Characteristics	Examples of Controlled Substances
Schedule I (CI)	No accepted medical use Highest potential for abuse Not available by prescription	Heroin and marijuana
Schedule II (CII)	High potential for abuse or misuse	Meperidine (Demerol®), methadone, morphine, oxycodone (OxyContin®), methylphenidate (Ritalin®)
Schedule III (CIII)	Potential risk for abuse, misuse, and dependence	Includes drug products that contain small quantities of controlled substances combined with other noncontrolled drugs such as acetaminophen and codeine (Tylenol and Codeine®) and hydrocodone with acetaminophen (Vicodin®)
Schedule IV (CIV)	Low potential for abuse and limited risk of dependence	Diazepam (Valium), lorazepam (Ativan), phenobarbital, and other sedatives and hypnotics
Schedule V (CV)	Low potential for abuse or misuse	Cough medications that contain a limited amount of codeine, antidiarrheal medications containing a limited amount of an opiate, and Lomotil®

the federal requirements for the OTC sales process and records. The pharmacist is responsible for making sure that these sales comply with state and federal laws and regulations for over-the-counter sales of Schedule V controlled substances.

Labeling of Controlled Substances

Federal law requires that packages of controlled substances (e.g., the drug manufacturer's packages) be labeled with a specific symbol to indicate that they are controlled substances.[7]

The controlled substance symbol must be prominent and sufficiently large so that it is clear that the drug is a controlled substance. FDA requires that the symbol is in the proper place and format on the prescription container label. The recognized symbol to indicate a controlled substance consists of a large letter "C" with the appropriate Roman numeral placed inside the "C" symbol. Federal law does not require that the pharmacy label patient prescription containers for controlled substance prescriptions with the federal controlled substance symbol.

**Federal Caution for Controlled Substances
Prescriptions Dispensed to Patients**

Caution: Federal law prohibits the transfer of this drug to
any person other than the patient for whom it was prescribed.

Federal law requires that pharmacies place a specific caution message on the container advising the patient that he or she may not give the controlled substance to any other person. The required statement is "Caution: Federal law prohibits the transfer of this drug to any person other than the patient for whom it was prescribed."

Prescribing, Dispensing, and Transferring Controlled Substances Prescriptions

Prescribing and dispensing of controlled substance prescriptions must comply with federal and state requirements. The prescriber is responsible for the legitimate prescribing and dispensing of controlled substances. The pharmacist has a corresponding responsibility to ensure that only legitimate controlled substance prescriptions are dispensed. Knowingly dispensing a controlled substance prescription that is not valid will subject the person to criminal and/or civil penalties and other adverse actions.

For a controlled substance prescription to be valid, it must be prescribed by a licensed prescriber for a legitimate medical purpose in the normal course of the prescriber's professional practice.[8] The prescribing practitioner must be registered with DEA (unless exempt from registration such as Public Health Service and Bureau of Prison physicians) and be licensed to prescribe controlled substances by the state in which the practitioner is operating. Pharmacists have a corresponding responsibility to dispense controlled substances pursuant to a valid prescription issued for a legitimate medical purpose in the course of the prescriber's practice. Pharmacists may, if necessary, verify the validity of controlled substance prescriptions. Prescribing a controlled substance or knowingly filling a controlled substance prescription in violation of the requirements may result in criminal or civil penalties for violation of the controlled substance laws.

Prescriptions for controlled substances may be issued only by a physician, dentist, podiatrist, veterinarian, or mid-level practitioner (such as a physician assistant or nurse) authorized under the state law, or other practitioners who are legally authorized to prescribe controlled substances in the state where the practitioner is licensed to practice and registered with the DEA unless exempt.

The authority of mid-level practitioners to prescribe controlled substances varies from state to state. In addition, mid-level practitioners may have prescribing authority limited to certain schedules of controlled substances or specific controlled substances. Mid-level practitioners may obtain DEA registration numbers to prescribe controlled substances if the state where they are licensed permits them to prescribe controlled substances. Examples of mid-level practitioners include physician assistants, nurse practitioners, optometrists, and a number of other practitioners.

Pharmacists may fill controlled substance prescriptions issued by out-of-state practitioners if allowed under state law or regulations. Because the state requirements vary, pharmacists in each state need to follow the different requirements. Generally, the prescribing practitioners must be authorized to prescribe controlled substances in the state where the prescriptions are issued. States have considerable differences in requirements for dispensing out-of-state prescriptions for controlled substances. States may place additional requirements on dispensing out-of-state controlled substance prescriptions. For example, the pharmacist may be required to use professional judgment regarding the validity of the prescription or to take reasonable steps to verify that the prescription is legitimate. In some states, the prescription must be dispensed within a certain time period such as within 30 days of issue by the prescriber.

Unless an oral prescription is permitted, controlled substance prescriptions are required to be written in ink or indelible pencil or typewritten and manually signed by the practitioner unless an exception is permitted. The practitioner's designated agent may prepare the prescription for the practitioner's signature. Controlled substance prescriptions must contain the following information:

▶ Date and signed on the date issued
▶ Patient's full name and address
▶ Practitioner's name, address, and DEA registration number
▶ Drug name, strength, dosage form, and quantity prescribed
▶ Directions for use
▶ Number of refills (if any) authorized
▶ Manual signature of prescriber (where an oral prescription is not permitted)

Schedule II prescriptions must be written and are not refillable. Pharmacists may only dispense Schedule II controlled substances pursuant to a written prescription signed by the practitioner. However, exceptions are allowed for an emergency and specific requirements must be met (21 Code of Federal Regulations 1306.11). In an emergency, the practitioner may provide an oral CII prescription to the pharmacist and the pharmacist may dispense the prescription. The quantity should be limited to the amount needed for the emergency. If the prescriber is not known to the pharmacist, a reasonable effort must be made to validate the prescriber. The prescribing practitioner must provide the original written signed

CII prescription to the pharmacist within 7 days with "authorization for emergency dispensing" written on the face of the prescription. The pharmacist must notify the DEA if the CII prescription is not received. In addition, prescribers may fax CII prescriptions to the pharmacy to assist patients. The original CII prescription must be presented to the pharmacist and the pharmacist must compare the original prescription to the facsimile prescription before dispensing. Both the faxed CII prescription and the original CII prescription must be kept by the pharmacy. Some states require Schedule II prescriptions to be written on special prescription forms (e.g., in Texas).

Federal regulations recognize three exceptions where the facsimile of the CII prescription may serve as the original prescription. These exceptions include a practitioner prescribing a Schedule II narcotic drug compounded for direct infusion administration to a patient, for a patient residing in a long-term care facility, or for a hospice patient.

Pharmacists are permitted to dispense part of the prescribed quantity of a Schedule II prescription if they are unable to dispense the full quantity. The partial quantity dispensed must be noted on the front of the prescription, and the remainder must be dispensed within 72 hours of the initial dispensing. If the remainder is not dispensed, the pharmacist is required to notify the prescriber, and a new prescription is required for further dispensing.[9]

Prescriptions for Schedule III, IV, and V controlled substances, including any renewal to authorize refills, may be communicated by the prescriber to the pharmacist in writing, orally, or by facsimile. Schedule CIII and IV prescriptions may only be refilled up to five times within 6 months after the date the prescription was issued by the prescriber. After 6 months, all unused refills for CIII and CIV prescriptions expire and a new prescription from the prescriber is required. Schedule V prescriptions may be refilled only as authorized by the prescriber. Pharmacists are required to record certain information on the back of the CIII–V prescription when it is refilled, including the pharmacist's initials, refill date, and amount of the controlled substance dispensed. Alternatively, pharmacies with computer systems may record the refill information electronically if the refill history information is retrievable online and the pharmacist verifies the accuracy of the computer prescription refill information. Pharmacies are required to maintain prescription and refill authorization information records for 2 years.

Transferring controlled substance prescriptions from one pharmacy to another is permitted under certain circumstances (**Box 5-1**). CII prescriptions are not transferable. However, federal law allows CIII–V prescriptions to be transferred from one pharmacy to another for refilling one time if the state permits the transfer under its laws. For pharmacies that have a real-time online computer system connecting their pharmacies, federal law allows CIII–V prescriptions to be transferred up to the maximum number of authorized refills. Federal regulations place a number of requirements on the transfer Schedule III, IV, and V controlled substance prescriptions. The prescription must be transferred between two licensed pharmacists and specific information must be written on the prescription being transferred, including "void" written on the face of the transferred prescription and the transfer date and name of the transferring pharmacist. The name, address, and DEA registration number of the pharmacy and the pharmacist receiving the prescription must be written on the back of the prescription. The receiving pharmacist must write transfer on the face of the prescription, and ensure that the following information is included: date of the original prescription; number of refills on original prescription; date of original dispensing; number of remaining refills with dates and locations of prior refills; the name, address, and DEA registration number of the transferring pharmacy; prescription number from the transferring pharmacy; and the name of the transferring pharmacist. The name,

---

Box 5-1
Transfer of Prescriptions for Schedule III, IV, and V
Controlled Substances

Federal Drug Enforcement Administration (DEA) allows the transfer of original prescription information for Schedules III, IV, and V controlled substances between pharmacies for refilling the prescription one time only, if allowed under state law with the following requirements:
- Transfer is communicated between two pharmacists
- Transferring pharmacist must:
  - Write "VOID" on the face of invalidated prescription
  - Record the name, address, and DEA number of the pharmacy receiving the transferred prescription and name of pharmacist receiving the prescription on back of the prescription
  - Record the transfer date and the transferring pharmacist name
- Receiving pharmacist must:
  - Write "transfer" on the face of the transferred prescription
  - Provide information required to be on a prescription and include:
    - Date original prescription issued
    - Number of refills on original prescription
    - Date the original prescription was dispensed
    - Number of valid refills remaining and dates and locations of prior refills
    - Pharmacy's name, address, DEA number, and prescription number from which the prescription information was transferred
    - Name of transferring pharmacist
    - Pharmacy's name, address, DEA number, and prescription number from which the prescription was originally filled

Pharmacies that electronically share a real time, online prescription database may transfer prescriptions up to the maximum refills permitted by law pursuant to the prescriber's authorization and must contain the information required for a valid prescription.

address, and DEA registration number of the original pharmacy must be included if it is different from the transferring pharmacy.

Federal law requires specific information to be on the patient's controlled substance prescription container label. The required information includes:

▶ Pharmacy name and address
▶ Prescription number
▶ Date of dispensing
▶ Patient name
▶ Prescribing practitioner name
▶ Drug name, strength, and quantity
▶ Directions for use

In addition, prescription labels for dispensed controlled substances must have the federal warning against providing the drug to any other persons. The statement must specifically state "Caution: Federal law prohibits the transfer of this drug to any person other than the patient for whom it was prescribed." (21 Code of Federal Regulations 290.5)

State laws require additional information on the patient's prescription container label, such as pharmacy phone number and remaining refills. Pharmacists will also add patient warning labels appropriate to the controlled substance based on the pharmacist's professional judgment. For example, controlled substances that are sleeping medications would be labeled with cautions that the medication causes drowsiness and not to drive or operate machinery.

Drug Enforcement Administration

The federal Drug Enforcement Administration (DEA), which is part of the Department of Justice, enforces the Controlled Substances Act to prevent diversion and abuse of controlled substances and regulated chemicals. DEA oversees the handling and distribution of controlled substances in compliance with the CSA. DEA does not routinely inspect pharmacies for controlled substance violations because state Boards of Pharmacy provide this oversight function. However, the DEA may investigate diversion of controlled substances from pharmacies through review of pharmacy prescription records, including investigations of forged controlled substance prescriptions and of persons attempting to obtain illegitimate controlled substance prescriptions through "doctor shopping." DEA advises pharmacists that they play an important role in the proper dispensing of controlled substances and prevention of abuse and diversion of controlled substances.

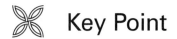 **Key Point**

The scope of DEA authority is determined by the CSA and is directed at enforcing the controlled substance laws and regulations and preventing diversion and abuse of controlled substances and drugs containing regulated chemicals.

Pharmacy DEA Registration

The CSA restricts access to controlled substances to persons and entities that are registered with DEA. Pharmacies, physicians, and others including prescribing practitioners; drug manufacturers; drug distributors; and drug importers and exporters must also have a DEA registration. A pharmacy's DEA registration permits the pharmacy to order and dispense controlled substances. DEA-registered pharmacies must comply with federal law and the state law where the pharmacy is located, including any more stringent state controlled substance laws and regulations.

To register with DEA, pharmacy owners must complete a DEA Form 224 called an "Application for New Registration." Pharmacies are required to renew their registration every 3 years. Each pharmacy location must have a separate DEA registration.

If a pharmacy moves to a new location or its address changes at the same location, the pharmacy must obtain a new DEA registration. Pharmacies must renew their DEA registration using DEA Form 224a.

Controlled Substances Ordering

Part of the CSA closed system for controlled substances is the requirement that CII controlled substances must be ordered using the DEA Official Order Form, known as DEA Form 222. Pharmacists are responsible for completing the DEA Form 222 to indicate the CII drug and quantity being ordered, and the form must be signed by the pharmacy's authorized pharmacist. These forms are also used by the pharmacist to document the quantity and date for received controlled substances on the pharmacy copy. Federal regulations require that the pharmacy keep the DEA Form 222s and that the forms have no alterations or changes. For CIII, IV, and V controlled substances, the pharmacy is not required to use a DEA Form 222. The pharmacy is permitted to use the drug purchasing invoice as the record of the order and the quantity received. Pharmacies are required to keep their controlled substance records so that they are ready to be provided for inspection by the DEA or the state Board of Pharmacy.

Security, Reporting of Thefts and Losses, and Recordkeeping

The CSA requires all DEA registrants, including pharmacies, to maintain physical and operational security measures to prevent theft and diversion of controlled substances. The type of security requirements depends on the DEA registrant. Drug manufacturers and distributors are required to store Schedule II substances in special vaults or safes and have electronic security for all storage areas. Pharmacies are permitted to keep controlled substances in locked cabinet or dispersed throughout the prescription drug stock. Practitioners are required to store all scheduled drugs in securely locked cabinet.

Pharmacies are required to keep complete, accurate, and up-to-date records for controlled substances that they purchase, receive, distribute, dispense, or discard. Schedule II records must be kept separately from CIII, IV, and V records. The comprehensive recordkeeping requirements permit controlled substances to be traced throughout their distribution and handling from their manufacture until dispensing to the patient. Federal law requires pharmacies to keep controlled substance records for a minimum of 2 years. States laws and regulations for controlled substances recordkeeping are variable, with a number of states requiring pharmacies to keep records for more than 2 years. State Boards of Pharmacy and DEA may review the records.

 # Key Point

Pharmacies are required to keep complete, accurate, and current records for controlled substances that they purchase, receive, distribute, dispense, or discard and immediately report any theft or significant loss to the DEA.

Pharmacies are required to immediately report any theft or significant loss of controlled substances to the DEA using DEA Form 106 "Report of Theft or Loss of Controlled Substances." A sample of the DEA Form 106 is available on the DEA Internet site at http://www.deadiversion.usdoj.gov/21cfr_reports/theft/106_blank. pdf. Small, repeated losses of controlled substances must be reported as they may indicate a significant problem. Pharmacies are also required to report any pharmacy break-in or armed robbery. Federal investigation of drug thefts or robberies of controlled substances is authorized under federal law if the replacement cost for the substances is $500 or higher, if a registrant is killed or suffers significant injury during the theft or robbery, and other reasons.[10] Many states require reporting of controlled substances thefts or losses.

Recordkeeping requirements are another significant part of the closed system controls for controlled substances. Pharmacies are required to maintain complete, current, and accurate records for all controlled substances that they purchase, receive, distribute, dispense, and discard. Federal law requires the pharmacy to keep controlled substance records for 2 years and have them readily available for DEA inspection if requested. State laws may require pharmacies to keep controlled substances records for a longer time period. State Boards of Pharmacy and DEA may review the records. Examples of records that must be kept include invoices or receipts for purchases of controlled substances; inventory records, including initial and biennial inventories; and records of any transfers of controlled substances between pharmacies. Other important controlled substance records that pharmacies must keep include the pharmacy's DEA registration certificate, the pharmacy's DEA order forms for CII drugs (DEA Form 222), prescription records for controlled substances, and records of any reports of any thefts or losses of controlled substances. Pharmacies must also keep records of any controlled substances that are destroyed or discarded using DEA Form 41. If any controlled substances are destroyed (such as when they have expired), pharmacies must complete and maintain a DEA Form 41.

Pharmacy controlled substance prescription records must be readily available and separated or marked to identify the different schedules of controlled substances for inspection by DEA or state authorities. Several options exist to meet these requirements, including 1) separate files for CII prescriptions, CIII through CV prescriptions, and prescriptions for non-controlled drugs dispensed; 2) two separate files with one for CII prescriptions, and a second for non-controlled drug prescriptions and CIII–V prescriptions marked with a large red "C" stamp; and 3) two separate files with one for all CII–V prescriptions with CIII–V marked with a red "C" stamp and a second file for prescriptions for non-controlled drug prescriptions. State laws may require one filing system over another.

State Prescription Monitoring Programs

Another means that states use to monitor controlled substances are prescription monitoring programs. These programs have been in use for many years. Initially, these programs existed in a small number of states and used manual systems that required pharmacies to submit copies of controlled substance prescriptions (such as triplicate prescription forms for CII prescriptions) to state controlled substance authorities. With expanded use of computer systems, these programs have developed into electronic monitoring programs that require pharmacies to submit their controlled substance prescription information to the designated state authority electronically on a periodic basis (e.g., once or twice a month or more frequently). More than 30 states have implemented these programs with more states considering or implementing these programs. The information that pharmacies provide to these programs include patient information, prescriber information, and pharmacy identification and prescription information such as the name and quantity of the controlled substance and the date the prescription was dispensed (**Box 5-2**).

These programs are used by states to identify potential diversion and abuse of prescription controlled substances drugs whether by the patient, pharmacy, or prescriber, and to identify potential patients that would benefit from drug abuse treatment programs. More information on controlled substances prescription monitoring programs is available from the website for the Alliance of States with Prescription Monitoring Programs at http://www.nascsa.org/monitoring.htm.

Restrictions on Sales of Products Containing Ephedrine, Pseudoephedrine, and Phenylpropanolamine

Some over-the-counter drug products are subject to additional restrictions under federal and state laws. These laws set restrictions on how the products are sold, limit the amount that a customer may purchase (e.g., in a single transaction, in a day, or over a 30-day period), require that the products be locked up or otherwise not available for public access without assistance, and require log books with details on the sales. These restrictions were enacted by states and Congress due to diversion of these legitimate OTC health care products for the illegal manufacture of methamphetamine. The products that are subject to these controls are common ingredients of cough and cold preparations available over-the-counter: pseudoephedrine, ephedrine, and phenylpropanolamine[11] (not available for sale in the United States).

In 2000, Congress enacted the Methamphetamine Anti-Proliferation Act to prevent diversion of OTC products containing pseudoephedrine by establishing a limited amount that could be purchased. In 2006, due to continuing concerns about OTC products being diverted for the illegal manufacture of methamphet-

---

Box 5-2
States with Prescription Monitoring Programs (2006)

Alabama	Iowa	New Mexico	Texas
California	Kentucky	New York	Utah
Colorado	Louisiana	Ohio	Vermont
Connecticut	Maine	Oklahoma	Virginia
Hawaii	Massachusetts	Pennsylvania	Washington
Idaho	Michigan	Rhode Island	West Virginia
Illinois	Mississippi	South Carolina	Wyoming
Indiana	Nevada	Tennessee	

amine, the federal government enacted the Combat Methamphetamine Epidemic Act (CMEA). The CMEA limits sales of products containing pseudoephedrine, ephedrine, and phenylpropanolamine to 3.6 grams daily. The law limits buyers to the purchase of 9 grams in a 30-day period, and requires that purchasers provide their photo identification and sign a log book with their name, address, and date and time of purchase. The log books may be used by law enforcement to identify violations of the law.

Many states have also enacted laws restricting the sale and purchase of these OTC products. A complete review of each state law is beyond the scope of this review. However, as with the federal CMEA, many state laws 1) restrict how the products are sold, 2) limit the amount that a retailer or pharmacy may sell and purchasers may buy, and 3) require purchasers to provide photo identification and sign a log book. Under some state laws, these products may only be sold in a pharmacy. Some states (e.g., Oklahoma) have scheduled these OTC drug products as Schedule V controlled substance or a Schedule III controlled substance (Oregon). In Oklahoma, only licensed pharmacists and pharmacy technicians are permitted to sell these OTC products and they must be stored behind the pharmacy counter. In Oregon, these CIII products require a prescription. The federal CMEA must be followed in all states, and, if the state is stricter, it must be followed. Pharmacy technicians will need to check with the pharmacist or the state Board of Pharmacy for the specific requirements applicable in a particular state.

Summary

Controlled substance drug products are subject to more stringent controls through federal and state laws and regulations because of their potential for misuse, abuse, diversion, and addiction. Controlled substances are divided into five different schedules based on their potential for misuse, abuse, and addiction. Controlled substance laws create a closed distribution system with recordkeeping to tightly regulate the distribution, prescribing, dispensing, and handling of these drug products. Requirements applicable to controlled substances include a requirement for pharmacies, prescribers, and others to register with the Drug Enforcement Administration (DEA); DEA registration numbers for the prescribers to prescribe controlled substances and for pharmacies to dispense controlled substances; special marks on drug manufacturer prescription containers to indicate controlled substances; limitations on prescribing, dispensing, and refilling these prescriptions; special labeling requirements for the patient's prescription container; and other requirements for storage, recordkeeping, distribution, and handling controlled substances.

The DEA requires the use of special forms to order controlled substances and to report the theft or loss of controlled substances. Controlled substances are subject to additional monitoring through prescription monitoring programs implemented by many states to collect information from pharmacies on the dispensing of these drugs. Federal and state laws have added special restrictions and requirements for sale of over-the-counter products containing pseudoephedrine, ephedrine, and phenylpropanolamine to prevent their diversion for illicit purposes.

References

1. See 21 U.S. Code Sections 801 et seq.
2. See Controlled Substances Act, 21 U.S. Code Section 802.
3. See 21 U.S. Code Section 811(c).
4. A complete list of controlled substances is available in Title 21 of the Code of Federal Regulations (21 CFR Part 1308).
5. See 21 Code of Federal Regulations Part 1308.15.
6. See 21 Code of Federal Regulations Section 1306.26.
7. See 21 Code of Federal Regulations Part 1302.
8. See 21 Code of Federal Regulations Section 1306.04(a).
9. See 21 Code of Federal Regulations Section 1306.13.
10. See Controlled Substances Registrant Protection Act of 1984.
11. Phenylpropanolamine was withdrawn from the market pursuant to FDA action; however, federal and state laws include phenylpropanolamine as one of the restricted substances.

Self-Assessment Questions

1. Why do controlled substances require more stringent controls by federal and state laws?
2. What is the CSA and what does it do?
3. A pharmacy, pharmacist, or physician must be registered with what federal agency to have access to controlled substances?
4. What process must a pharmacy follow if a controlled substance is stolen or lost from the pharmacy?
5. What is the CMEA and what does it do?

Chapter 6

State Laws and Regulations for Pharmacy Practice

Chapter Outline

Learning Objectives

1. Describe how the state pharmacy laws typically define the role of pharmacy technicians.
2. List the general state Board of Pharmacy functions.
3. Identify the different types of state pharmacy licenses.
4. List the most common requirements for pharmacist licensure applicants.
5. List the common regulatory requirements for pharmacy technicians.
6. Discuss the general difference between registration and licensure.
7. Describe the common requirements for pharmacy technician licensure and registration.
8. Discuss the different applications of certification of pharmacy technicians.
9. Define the application of pharmacy technician ratios under pharmacy practice laws.
10. Describe the regulation of permitted acts and responsibilities of pharmacy technicians.

Practice of Pharmacy

This chapter discusses the major components of the state pharmacy laws and regulations, commonly known as the state pharmacy practice acts in relation to pharmacy technicians. Pharmacy practice acts include provisions affecting pharmacies, pharmacists, pharmacy technicians, and the requirements to practice pharmacy. State pharmacy practice acts and regulations are generally similar. However, the particular requirements are likely to vary from state to state. Because the pharmacy laws and regulations vary depending on the state, the state Boards of Pharmacy for each state are a resource for specific information for each state.

A starting point for considering pharmacy practice laws and regulations is the definition of the "practice of pharmacy." State pharmacy laws generally include a definition of the "practice of pharmacy." The definition of the practice of pharmacy describes the scope of professional acts that pharmacists are permitted to perform as they practice pharmacy in that particular state. Pharmacy technicians assist pharmacists in the practice of pharmacy with the nondiscretionary and nonjudgmental tasks that do not require a pharmacist's professional judgment and are not restricted to pharmacists only. Pharmacists are generally permitted to perform similar responsibilities in each state. Some states permit pharmacists to engage in additional professional duties such as collaborative practice with physicians and the administration of vaccinations. Pharmacists practicing in each state will be familiar with their permitted scope of practice. The National Association of Boards of Pharmacy (NABP) Model Act provides a model definition of the "practice of pharmacy."

 Key Point

Pharmacy technicians assist pharmacists in the practice of pharmacy with the nondiscretionary and nonjudgmental tasks that do not require a pharmacist's professional judgment and are not restricted to pharmacists only (**Box 6-1**).

In some states, the definition of the practice of pharmacy may include additional items such as modifying drug therapy according to written protocols. In Mississippi, the Board of Pharmacy's definition of pharmacy practice allows pharmacists to initiate or modify drug therapy in accord with written guidelines or protocols.

Mississippi Definition of Practice of Pharmacy

"Practice of pharmacy" shall mean a health care service that includes, but is not limited to, the compounding, dispensing, and labeling of

---

Box 6-1
NABP Definition of the Practice of Pharmacy

The "Practice of Pharmacy" means the interpretation, evaluation, and implementation of Medical Orders; the Dispensing of Prescription Drug Orders; participation in Drug and Device selection; Drug Administration; Drug Regimen Reviews; the Practice of Telepharmacy within and across state lines; Drug or Drug-related research; the provision of Patient Counseling and the provision of those acts or services necessary to provide Pharmaceutical Care in all areas of patient care, including Primary Care and Collaborative Pharmacy Practice; and the responsibility for Compounding and Labeling of Drugs and Devices (except Labeling by a Manufacturer, repackager, or Distributor of Non-Prescription Drugs and commercially packaged Legend Drugs and Devices), proper and safe storage of Drugs and Devices, and maintenance of proper records for them.

---

drugs or devices; interpreting and evaluating prescriptions; administering and distributing drugs and devices; the compounding, dispensing and labeling of drugs and devices; maintaining prescription drug records; advising and consulting concerning therapeutic values, content, hazards and uses of drugs and devices; initiating or modifying of drug therapy in accordance with written guidelines or protocols previously established and approved by the board; selecting drugs; participating in drug utilization reviews; storing prescription drugs and devices; ordering lab work in accordance with written guidelines or protocols as defined by paragraph (jj) of this section; providing pharmacotherapeutic consultations; supervising supportive personnel and such other acts, services, operations or transactions necessary or incidental to the conduct of the foregoing. (Mississippi Code Section 73-21-73)

In Oregon, the pharmacist's scope of practice definition allows pharmacists to administer vaccines and other drugs if permitted.

Oregon Definition of Practice of Pharmacy
The "practice of pharmacy" means the interpretation and evaluation of prescription orders; the compounding, dispensing, labeling of drugs and devices (except labeling by a manufacturer, packer or distributor of nonprescription drugs and commercially packaged legend drugs and devices); the administering of vaccines and immunizations pursuant to Oregon Statute 689.645; the administering of drugs and devices to the extent permitted under Oregon Statute 689.655; the participa-

tion in drug selection and drug utilization reviews; the proper and safe storage of drugs and devices and the maintenance of proper records therefor; the responsibility for advising, where necessary or where regulated, of therapeutic values, content, hazards and use of drugs and devices; the monitoring of therapeutic response or adverse effect to drug therapy; and the offering or performing of those acts, services, operations or transactions necessary in the conduct, operation, management and control of pharmacy. (Oregon Statute Section 689.015)

Pharmacy technicians work under the direction and supervision of pharmacists and may perform the tasks permitted under state law. State pharmacy laws and regulations distinguish between the tasks and responsibilities that pharmacists perform and those that pharmacy technicians are permitted to perform. Pharmacy technicians are not permitted to perform pharmacy practice responsibilities that require the professional judgment, education, and training of a licensed pharmacist. For example, the Iowa pharmacy law states that a "person shall not engage in the practice of pharmacy in this state without a license" and that the "license shall be identified as a pharmacist license." In general, pharmacy technicians are permitted to perform nonjudgmental and nondiscretionary tasks under the pharmacist's supervision. In addition, most states define the pharmacy technician's permitted tasks.

 Key Point

Pharmacy technicians work under the direction and supervision of pharmacists and may perform the tasks permitted under state law. State pharmacy laws and regulations distinguish between the tasks and responsibilities that pharmacists perform and those that pharmacy technicians are permitted to perform under the pharmacist's supervision.

Pharmacies and Pharmacists

The state Board of Pharmacy is the primary state agency responsible for regulating the practice of pharmacy in each state, including requirements for pharmacies, pharmacists, pharmacy interns, and pharmacy technicians. The state Boards of Pharmacy are generally established through the state pharmacy practice laws. These state laws give the state Boards of Pharmacy regulatory authority over a number of areas such as licensing pharmacies and pharmacists, regulating pharmacy technicians, promulgating rules and regulations, and instituting disciplinary actions against pharmacies, pharmacists, pharmacy technicians, and pharmacy interns (**Box 6-2**, page 74).

Pharmacy Licensure

State pharmacy laws and regulations give state Boards of Pharmacy authority to license pharmacies and to set the requirements and specifications for pharmacy licensure. Every state requires pharmacies to have a state-issued pharmacy license or permit in order to operate the pharmacy. The NABP Model State Pharmacy Act provides an example of a pharmacy licensure law (**Box 6-3**). Requirements for pharmacy licensure include many items such as required equipment, references, hours of operation, security, and having a licensed pharmacist on duty while the pharmacy is open. State Boards of Pharmacy conduct pharmacy inspections to verify that the pharmacy meets the licensure requirements and also perform periodic pharmacy inspections at other times. Pharmacies are required to post their license or permit in the pharmacy. Pharmacies that do not have valid current licenses or permits are in violation of state law and subject to fines or penalties.

State pharmacy laws define a pharmacy, require pharmacies to be licensed, and require that all areas where prescription drugs are dispensed and pharmacist services are provided be restricted to pharmacists and authorized pharmacy personnel. For example, Iowa law defines a pharmacy license as being issued to a pharmacy or another location where prescription drugs or devices are dispensed pursuant to a prescription.[1] Iowa law also prohibits a person from operating a pharmacy without a license.

> A person shall not establish, conduct, or maintain a pharmacy in this state without a license. The license shall be identified as a pharmacy license. A pharmacy license . . . may be further identified as a hospital pharmacy license.[2]

Another example is California where they define a pharmacy in terms of the area where the profession of pharmacy is practiced and where prescription drugs are stored and dispensed. California law states:

> Pharmacy means an area, place, or premises licensed by the board in which the profession of pharmacy is practiced and where prescriptions are compounded. Pharmacy includes, but is not limited to, any area, place, or premises described in a license issued by the board wherein controlled substances, dangerous drugs, or dangerous devices are stored, possessed, prepared, manufactured, derived, compounded, or repackaged, and from which the controlled substances, dangerous drugs, or dangerous devices are furnished, sold, or dispensed at retail.[3]

State pharmacy laws also define hospital pharmacies and restrict access to pharmacists, pharmacy technicians, and other appropriate persons. For example, California law states:

> No person other than a pharmacist, an intern pharmacist, a pharmacy technician, an authorized officer of the law, a person authorized to prescribe, a registered nurse, a licensed vocational nurse, a person who enters the pharmacy for purposes of receiving consultation from a pharmacist, or a person authorized by the pharmacist in charge to perform clerical, inventory control, housekeeping, delivery, maintenance, or similar functions relating to the pharmacy shall be permitted in that area, place, or premises described in the license issued by the board to a licensed hospital wherein controlled substances, dangerous drugs, or dangerous devices are stored, possessed, prepared, manufactured, derived, compounded, dispensed, or repackaged.[4]

Many state pharmacy laws prevent the use of the word pharmacy, pharmacist, or similar words in building signs without a pharmacy license. California law is an example.

> No building shall have upon it or displayed within it or affixed to or used in connection with it a sign bearing the word or words "Pharmacist," "Pharmacy," "Apothecary," "Drugstore," "Druggist," "Drugs," "Medicine," "Medicine Store," "Drug Sundries," "Remedies," or any word or words of similar or like import; or the characteristic symbols of pharmacy; or the characteristic prescription sign (Rx) or similar design, unless there is upon or within the building a pharmacy holding a license issued by the board pursuant to Section 4110.[5]

Many states have more than one category of pharmacy license. The different licensure categories that states may identify include retail, community, institution-

---

Box 6-2
General State Board of Pharmacy Functions

- Licensing pharmacies
- Licensing pharmacists
- Promulgating rules and regulations
- Inspecting pharmacies
- Investigating complaints and violations of the laws and regulations
- Disciplining pharmacies, pharmacists, and pharmacy technicians for violations

---

Box 6-3
Licensure of Pharmacies

(a) The following Persons located within this State, and the following Persons located outside this State that provide services to patients within this State, shall be licensed by the Board of Pharmacy and shall annually renew their license with the Board:
   (1) Persons engaged in the Practice of Pharmacy;
   (2) Persons engaged in the Manufacture, production, sale, or Distribution of Drugs or Devices;
   (3) Pharmacies where Drugs or Devices are Dispensed, or Pharmaceutical Care is provided; and
   (4) Pharmacy Benefits Managers.

Source: NABP Model State Pharmacy Act, August 2006.

---

al, hospital, nuclear, mail order, and long-term care. Some states use categories for pharmacies such as special or limited-use pharmacies and sterile compounding pharmacies. Another category used by states is non-resident pharmacies, which are pharmacies located outside of a state. Most states require pharmacies that are located in another state (i.e., non-resident pharmacies) to be licensed in the state if they mail, ship, dispense, or deliver prescription drugs to residents of the state. Wisconsin law provides an example.[6]

(1) No pharmacy that is in another state may ship, mail, or otherwise deliver a prescribed drug or device to persons in this state unless the pharmacy is licensed under sub. (2).
(2) The board shall issue a license to a pharmacy that is located outside this state if the pharmacy does all of the following:
   (a) Applies on a form provided by the board that shows all of the following:
      1. The location of the pharmacy.
      2. The name and address of the person holding title and ownership control of the location.
      3. The name of the managing pharmacist of the pharmacy.
   (b) Submits a statement in a form prescribed by the board from the owner of the pharmacy or, if the pharmacy is not a sole proprietorship, from the managing pharmacist of the pharmacy that indicates that the owner or managing pharmacist, whichever is applicable, knows the laws relating to the practice of pharmacy in this state.
   (c) Submits evidence satisfactory to the board that it is licensed in the state in which it is located.

States require the pharmacy to identify the pharmacist who will be in charge of the pharmacy as one of the requirements to obtain the pharmacy permit or license. For example, Oregon requires the pharmacy registration application to identify the pharmacist in charge.[7]

> Applications for certificates of registration shall include the following information about the proposed drug outlet:
>
> (a)   Ownership;
>
> (b)   Location;
>
> (c)   Identity of pharmacist licensed to practice in the state, who shall be the pharmacist in charge of the drug outlet, where one is required by this chapter, and such further information as the board may deem necessary; and [other requirements omitted.]

State pharmacy licensure is an example of the extensive state Board of Pharmacy oversight and regulation of the practice of pharmacy. Pharmacy technicians need to be aware that pharmacies are licensed by state Boards of Pharmacy and that access to the prescription area of pharmacies is restricted to certain persons such as pharmacists, pharmacy interns, pharmacy technicians, and other appropriate persons (e.g., nurses in a hospital pharmacy, state Board of Pharmacy inspectors). The public is not allowed in a pharmacy.

Pharmacist Licensure

State Boards of Pharmacy have authority over the licensure of pharmacists practicing pharmacy in the state. State pharmacy laws make it unlawful for anyone to practice pharmacy without a license. State pharmacy laws and regulations also establish the requirements for pharmacist licensure. These requirements are generally similar from state to state. Most states require pharmacist licensure applicants to graduate from an approved college or school of pharmacy, complete specified internship requirements, and successfully pass the pharmacist licensure and law examinations. For example, Iowa law places the following requirements on pharmacist licensure:[8]

1. Be a graduate of a school or college of pharmacy or of a department of pharmacy of a university recognized and approved by the board.
2. File proof, satisfactory to the board, of internship for a period of time fixed by the board.
3. Pass an examination prescribed by the board.

A nationwide shortage of pharmacists in the United States was identified in 1998, with the shortage varying from state to state.[9] The shortage results primarily from an increased demand for pharmacist services coupled with the difficulty of rapidly increasing the supply of pharmacists. At least one state, California, enacted a law to review the shortage and make recommendations to alleviate the pharmacist shortage. The law states:

> The Joint Committee on Boards, Commissions, and Consumer Protection shall review the state's shortage of pharmacists and make recommendations on a course of action to alleviate the shortage, including, but not limited to, a review of the current California pharmacist licensure examination.[10]

Graduates from foreign pharmacy schools are permitted to seek pharmacist licensure but must meet additional requirements. For example, foreign pharmacy graduates must take a foreign pharmacy graduate equivalency examination and an examination to assess competency in the English language unless exempt from this requirement.

Board of Pharmacy Rules and Regulations

State pharmacy laws give state Boards of Pharmacy authority to adopt rules and regulations for the practice of pharmacy. State Boards of Pharmacy adopt rules and regulations related to a number of legal requirements such as pharmacist licensure, dispensing of prescriptions, pharmacy licensure, and the scope of pharmacy practice. For example, Oregon law gives the Board of Pharmacy authority to adopt necessary rules.[11] The National Association of Boards of Pharmacy Model Rules provides an example of a law giving Boards of Pharmacy rulemaking authority (**Box 6-4**).

State pharmacy laws give state Boards authority to regulate pharmacy technicians through adoption of necessary rules and regulations. For example, New Jersey law gives the Board power and authority necessary to enforce the rules and regulations of the Board, including regulation over the training, qualifications, and conduct of pharmacy technicians. New Jersey law states:[12]

> The board shall have those other duties, powers and authority as may be necessary to the enforcement of this act and to the enforcement of rules and regulations of the board, which may include, but not be limited to, the following:
>
> (1) The determination and issuance of standards, recognition and approval of degree programs of schools and colleges of pharmacy whose graduates shall be eligible for licensure in this State, and

the specifications and enforcement of requirements for practical training, including internships;

(2) The registration of externs, interns, pharmacy preceptors and pharmacy technicians;

(3) The regulation of the training, qualifications and conduct of applicants, externs, interns, pharmacy preceptors and pharmacy technicians.

Another example is New Mexico. The pharmacy practice law gives the Board of Pharmacy authority to adopt, amend, or repeal regulations; regulate examination requirements for pharmacists and pharmacist licenses; regulate pharmacy technicians; regulate licensing of pharmacies; and regulate numerous other areas.[13]

The board shall:

(1) adopt, amend or repeal rules and regulations necessary to carry out the provisions of the Pharmacy Act in accordance with the provisions of the Uniform Licensing Act;

(2) provide for examinations of applicants for licensure as pharmacists;

(3) provide for the issuance and renewal of licenses for pharmacists;

(4) require and establish criteria for continuing education as a condition of renewal of licensure for pharmacists;

(5) provide for the issuance and renewal of licenses for pharmacist interns and for their training, supervision and discipline;

(6) provide for the licensing of retail pharmacies, nonresident pharmacies, wholesale drug distributors, drug manufacturers, hospital pharmacies, nursing home drug facilities, industrial and public health clinics and all places where dangerous drugs are stored, distributed, dispensed or administered and provide for the inspection of the facilities and activities;

(7) enforce the provisions of all laws of the state pertaining to the practice of pharmacy and the manufacture, production, sale or distribution of drugs or cosmetics and their standards of strength and purity;

(8) conduct hearings upon charges relating to the discipline of a registrant or licensee or the denial, suspension or revocation of a registration or a license in accordance with the Uniform Licensing Act;

(9) cause the prosecution of any person violating the Pharmacy Act, the New Mexico Drug, Device and Cosmetic Act or the Controlled Substances Act;

(10) keep a record of all proceedings of the board;

(11) make an annual report to the governor;

(12) appoint and employ, in the board's discretion, a qualified person who is not a member of the board to serve as executive director and define the executive director's duties and responsibilities; except that the power to deny, revoke or suspend any license or registration authorized by the Pharmacy Act shall not be delegated by the board;

(13) appoint and employ inspectors necessary to enforce the provisions of all acts under the administration of the board, which inspectors shall be pharmacists and have all the powers and duties of peace officers;

(14) provide for other qualified employees necessary to carry out the provisions of the Pharmacy Act;

(15) have the authority to employ a competent attorney to give advice and counsel in regard to any matter connected with the duties of the board, to represent the board in any legal proceedings and to aid in the enforcement of the laws in relation to the pharmacy profession and to fix the compensation to be paid to the attorney; provided, however, that the attorney shall be compensated from the money of the board, including that provided for in Section 61-11-19;

(16) register and regulate qualifications, training and permissible activities of pharmacy technicians.

Although pharmacy laws vary, each state has laws giving the Board of Pharmacy (or the state agency that regulates pharmacy practice) the authority to adopt rules and regulations and regulate the practice of pharmacy in the state.

Box 6-4
State Board Rulemaking Authority

The Board of Pharmacy shall make, adopt, amend, and repeal such rules as may be deemed necessary by the Board from time to time for the proper administration and enforcement of this Act. Such rules shall be promulgated in accordance with the procedures specified in the Administrative Procedures Act of this State.

Source: NABP Model State Pharmacy Act, August, 2006.

Investigations and Discipline

State pharmacy laws give state Boards of Pharmacy disciplinary authority over pharmacies, pharmacists, pharmacy technicians, and other aspects of pharmacy practice. State Board of Pharmacy authority includes inspections, investigations, and disciplinary actions for violating pharmacy laws and regulations and engaging in unprofessional conduct. An example of language giving state Boards of Pharmacy authority to take disciplinary and enforcement actions is provided in **Appendix 6-1** at the end of this chapter showing the NABP Model Act "Discipline" provision.

California law provides another example. California law gives the Board of Pharmacy authority to take action against any person holding a license issued by the Board and found guilty of unprofessional conduct, and lists the types of unprofessional conduct.[14] The Board has authority to discipline for a number of actions such as incompetence, gross negligence, and wrongfully providing controlled substances. The following is a summary of the types of matters for which the California Board of Pharmacy has authority to take disciplinary action.

> The board shall take action against any holder of a license who is guilty of unprofessional conduct or whose license has been procured by fraud or misrepresentation or issued by mistake. Unprofessional conduct shall include, but is not limited to, any of the following:

- Gross immorality
- Incompetence
- Gross negligence
- Clearly excessive furnishing of controlled substances
- Any act involving moral turpitude, dishonesty, fraud, deceit, or corruption, whether the act is committed in the course of relations as a licensee or otherwise, and whether the act is a felony or misdemeanor or not
- Knowingly making or signing any certificate or other document that falsely represents the existence or nonexistence of a state of facts
- Administering any controlled substance by the person, or the use of any dangerous drug or of alcoholic beverages to the extent or in a manner as to be dangerous or injurious to oneself, to a person holding a license under this chapter, or to any other person or to the public, or to the extent that the use impairs the ability of the person to conduct with safety to the public the practice authorized by the license
- Unless authorized by law, knowingly selling, furnishing, giving away, or administering, or offering to sell, furnish, give away, or administer, any controlled substance to an addict

- Violating any of the statutes of this state, of any other state, or of the United States regulating controlled substances and dangerous drugs
- Conviction of more than one misdemeanor or any felony involving the use, consumption, or self-administration of any dangerous drug or alcoholic beverage, or any combination of those substances
- Conviction of a crime substantially related to the qualifications, functions, and duties of a licensee under the pharmacy law
- Conviction including a guilty plea of a violation state or federal controlled substances or prescription drug laws is conclusive evidence of unprofessional conduct duties of a licensee under this chapter
- Revocation, suspension, or discipline by another state of a license to practice pharmacy, operate a pharmacy, or do any other act for which a license is required by this chapter
- Engaging in any conduct that undermines a board investigation

California pharmacy law also addresses acts that constitute unprofessional conduct for a pharmacist:[15]

Unprofessional conduct for a pharmacist may include any of the following:

(a) Acts or omissions that involve, in whole or in part, the inappropriate exercise of his or her education, training, or experience as a pharmacist, whether or not the act or omission arises in the course of the practice of pharmacy or the ownership, management, administration, or operation of a pharmacy or other entity licensed by the board.

(b) Acts or omissions that involve, in whole or in part, the failure to exercise or implement his or her best professional judgment or corresponding responsibility with regard to the dispensing or furnishing of controlled substances, dangerous drugs, or dangerous devices, or with regard to the provision of services.

(c) Acts or omissions that involve, in whole or in part, the failure to consult appropriate patient, prescription, and other records pertaining to the performance of any pharmacy function.

(d) Acts or omissions that involve, in whole or in part, the failure to fully maintain and retain appropriate patient-specific information pertaining to the performance of any pharmacy function.

Each state has its own disciplinary authority law. The state Board of Pharmacy is a resource for complete information on disciplinary law, acts that constitute violations, and possible penalties for the state where the pharmacy technician is employed.

If a Board of Pharmacy determines that a violation of pharmacy law or regulation has occurred, the Board will notify the person or pharmacy involved of the violation. Depending on the Board's decision, the violation may be handled through informal discussions with the Board to resolve the matter, or the matter may proceed to an administrative disciplinary hearing before the Board. In some states, the Board has authority to issue a warning or notice of deficiency and order that corrective actions to fix the violation be taken in a certain time period.

If the violation is handled through an administrative hearing before the Board of Pharmacy, the Board considers evidence such as documents and testimony from the person (e.g., pharmacy, pharmacist, intern pharmacist, or pharmacy technician) charged with the violation. The pharmacy, pharmacist, pharmacy technician, or pharmacy intern may be represented by an attorney at the Board hearing and at other meetings with the Board. At the conclusion of the hearing, the Board will make a decision regarding the violation and the discipline. The Board may take different disciplinary actions such as issuing fines and penalties, suspending or revoking a license or registration, or imposing other requirements or penalties. The amount of the monetary penalties that state Boards may impose vary from state to state and for the different types of violations.

State Boards of Pharmacy have disciplinary authority, oversight, and enforcement power over the practice of pharmacy from licensure and registration requirements for pharmacy technicians, pharmacists, and pharmacies to requirements for prescription dispensing, pharmacy recordkeeping, and any other aspect of pharmacy practice. Knowledge of the applicable state pharmacy laws and regulations covering pharmacy technicians is important. The state Boards of Pharmacy are a resource for this information. See Appendix 6-2.

Pharmacy Technicians

Pharmacy technicians are an integral part of pharmacy practice. With the increasing role of pharmacy technicians, many states have enacted laws and adopted regulations establishing requirements that pharmacy technicians must meet to be able to assist pharmacists. These requirements vary from state to state. However, similarities exist. This section will discuss the common types of pharmacy technician requirements including registration or licensure (or similar requirements such as a certificate or permit), continuing education, permitted tasks and responsibilities, prohibited conduct, and penalties for violations of laws and regulations. This section will also discuss specific requirements to obtain registration or licensure such as a minimum age to work as a pharmacy technician or trainee, education and training, examinations, certification examinations, continuing education, and criminal background checks (**Box 6-5**).

Box 6-5
Common Regulatory Requirements for Pharmacy Technicians

- Registration or licensure (or certificate or permit in some state)
- Minimum age
- Training and education
- Examinations
- Certification
- Continuing education
- Criminal background checks
- Permitted tasks and responsibilities
- Pharmacy technician-to-pharmacist ratios
- Prohibited conduct
- Penalties

Progressively more states have enacted laws and regulations to require pharmacy technicians to be registered or licensed (or have a certificate or a permit) as a condition of being permitted to work in a pharmacy and perform pharmacy technician duties and to establish permitted tasks, prohibited conduct, and other requirements. Each state that regulates pharmacy technicians has its own laws and regulations, and pharmacy technicians will need to know the requirements for their particular state.

Registration and Licensure

Many state Boards of Pharmacy require pharmacy technicians to be registered, licensed, or have a permit or certificate as a condition of working as a pharmacy technician (**Box 6-6**). Nearly three-fourths of the states require pharmacy technicians to be licensed or registered. The majority of states require pharmacy technician registration rather than licensure. These requirements allow states to monitor individuals working in pharmacies as pharmacy technicians, assure that they meet certain requirements (such as age and education and training requirements), regulate the tasks that pharmacy technicians may perform, and allow for disciplinary actions against pharmacy technicians for violations of state pharmacy laws and regulations, including loss of licensure or registration if appropriate.

 # Key Point

Many state Boards of Pharmacy require pharmacy technicians to be registered, licensed, or have a permit or certificate as a condition of working as a pharmacy technician.

Box 6-6
Pharmacy Technician Licensure,
Registration, Permits, or Certificates

Licensure: Alaska, Arizona, California, Oregon, Rhode Island, Utah, and Wyoming

Registration or Permit: Alabama, Arkansas, Connecticut, Idaho, Illinois, Iowa, Kansas, Louisiana, Maine, Maryland, Massachusetts, Minnesota, Mississippi, Missouri, Montana, Nebraska, Nevada, New Hampshire, New Jersey, New Mexico, North Carolina, North Dakota, Oklahoma (permit), Puerto Rico, South Carolina, South Dakota, Tennessee, Texas, Vermont, Virginia, Washington (pharmacy assistants), West Virginia, and Wyoming

Certificate: Indiana

Certification: Washington

Registration is a process under which a state requires persons seeking to engage in certain activities to enroll or register to engage in a particular function. The state maintains a list of persons granted registration and usually requires that the registration be renewed on a periodic basis. Registration may have fewer eligibility criteria than licensure, and generally an examination is not required. However, for pharmacy technicians, there may be less distinction between the requirements for registration and licensure.

Generally, licensure is the process by which a state grants a license to a person to allow that person to work in a particular profession. Many professions require persons to be licensed. The purpose of licensure is to assure that the person is competent to provide the professional services. Pharmacists, nurses, lawyers, psychologists, and public accountants are examples of professions that require licensure. Licensure typically has higher requirements than registration, including completion of specific educational degrees, passing a specific professional examination, and other training and experience. For example, pharmacists are required to graduate from an approved school or college of pharmacy, pass the pharmacist licensure examinations, complete required experiential or intern training, and fulfill other requirements.

 # Key Point

Registration requires persons seeking to engage in certain activities to enroll or register to engage in the permitted activities or participate in a particular function. *Licensure is granted by the state to allow a person to work in a particular profession.*

The requirements for pharmacy technician licensure or registration or other status such as a certificate or permit depend on the specific state laws and regulations. Whether a state requires registration, licensure, a permit, or a certificate, the requirements may be more similar than different. Similar requirements may result in registration in one state and licensure in another state. Regardless of whether a state requires licensure, registration, or another required status, pharmacy technicians must meet the requirements to work as a pharmacy technician in the state. State Boards of Pharmacy have information available to inform pharmacy technicians of the requirements. See **Appendix 6-2** for information on contacting Boards of Pharmacy.

State Board Authority for Licensure or Registration

State pharmacy laws give state Boards of Pharmacy authority to license, register, or set other requirements for pharmacy technicians. Although most states use the terms licensure and registration, some states require pharmacy technicians to have a permit or certificate. For example, Indiana issues a certificate to an individual who meets the pharmacy technician requirements. In this instance, a certificate is similar in effect to registration and is not the same as passing a pharmacy technician certification exam. Certification examinations for pharmacy technicians are discussed in another section.

A number of states, including Alaska, Arizona, California, Oregon, Rhode Island, Utah, and Wyoming, require pharmacy technicians to be licensed. Alaska pharmacy law gives the Board of Pharmacy the power to license and regulate the training, qualifications, and employment of pharmacy technicians.[16] Alaska pharmacy law, as an example, states:

(a) The board is responsible for the control and regulation of the practice of pharmacy.

(b) In order to fulfill its responsibilities, the board has the powers necessary for implementation and enforcement of this chapter, including the power to ... license and regulate the training, qualifications, and employment of pharmacy interns and pharmacy technicians.

Examples of other state laws with similar effects include the following. Arizona pharmacy law sets the requirements for the Board of Pharmacy to license pharmacy technicians.[17] California pharmacy law states that no person shall act as a pharmacy technician without first being licensed by the Board as a pharmacy technician.[18] Oregon pharmacy law provides that the state Board of Pharmacy is responsible for the control and regulation of the practice of pharmacy in the state, including the licensing of pharmacy technicians.[19] Rhode Island pharmacy law gives the Board authority to establish qualifications for licensure of pharmacy technicians, pharmacists, and pharmacy interns.[20] Utah law requires a license to practice as a pharmacy technician.[21] Wyoming pharmacy law requires pharmacy technicians to register and become licensed.[22]

Many state pharmacy laws give the state Boards of Pharmacy authority to register pharmacy technicians. For example, Minnesota pharmacy law states that the Board of Pharmacy has the power and the duty to register pharmacy technicians.[23] Minnesota pharmacy law contains the following language pertinent to pharmacy technicians:

> The Board of Pharmacy shall have the power and it shall be its duty . . . to register pharmacy technicians; and to perform such other duties and exercise such other powers as the provisions of the act may require.

Other states have similar laws. Montana pharmacy law requires the Board of Pharmacy to regulate the practice of pharmacy, including the training, qualifications, employment, and registration of pharmacy technicians.[24] New Jersey law states that the Board is responsible for the control and regulation of the practice of pharmacy, including the registration, training, qualifications, and conduct of pharmacy technicians.[25] In Oklahoma, the pharmacy laws states no person shall serve as a pharmacy technician without first procuring a permit from the Board.[26] West Virginia law provides—as the reason for registering pharmacy technicians—that it is in the best interests of the public health, safety, and welfare that licensed pharmacists in this state be assisted with or relieved of certain tasks so that the pharmacist may counsel patients and improve pharmaceutical care and therapeutic outcomes, and that the Board shall recognize and register pharmacy technicians.[27] West Virginia law provides an example of state law referring to the role of pharmacy technicians assisting pharmacists in conjunction with the registration requirements.

(a)   The Legislature finds that it is in the best interests of the public health, safety and welfare that licensed pharmacists in this state be assisted with or relieved of certain tasks so that the pharmacist may counsel patients, improve pharmaceutical care and therapeutic outcomes. To achieve this aim, the board shall recognize and register pharmacy technicians.

(b)   On or after the first day of July, one thousand nine hundred ninety-six, any person practicing as a pharmacy technician in this state shall be registered with the board of pharmacy pursuant to the provisions of this section.

(c)   In order to become registered as pharmacy technicians in this state, individuals shall:

(1) Be at least eighteen years old;

(2) Be a high school graduate or its equivalent;

(3) Present to the board satisfactory evidence that he or she is of good moral character, is not addicted to alcohol or controlled substances and is free of any felony convictions; and

(4) Satisfactorily complete a board-approved pharmacy technician training program.

(d) The pharmacy technician training program and its curriculum shall be designed to train individuals to perform nonprofessional functions as described in legislative rules promulgated in accordance with the provisions of article three, chapter twenty-nine-a of this code.

(e) Pharmacy technicians shall be identified by a name tag and designation as pharmacy technician while working in a pharmacy within this state. A ratio of no more than four pharmacy technicians per on-duty pharmacist operating in any outpatient, mail order or institutional pharmacy shall be maintained.

Whether the state requires licensure or registration or issues a permit or certificate, pharmacy technicians may contact the state Board of Pharmacy for information on the requirements to work as a pharmacy technician. See Appendix 6-2 for a list of the state Boards of Pharmacy and the contact information.

Requirements for Pharmacy Technician Licensure or Registration

State pharmacy laws or regulations set the particular requirements that the pharmacy technicians must meet to obtain a license, registration, permit, or certificate. Although the requirements vary from state to state, most states require a minimum age, good moral character, high school graduation or the equivalent, and training. The common elements in most states include:

▶ Minimum age

▶ Good moral character

▶ High school graduation or an equivalent education degree or certificate

▶ Education and training programs

▶ Passing a pharmacy technician examination, which may require Board approval

 Key Point

State pharmacy laws or regulations set the particular requirements that the pharmacy technicians must meet to obtain a license, registration, permit, or certificate.

Some states have requirements for pharmacy technician trainees and pharmacy technicians. Arizona is an example of such a state.[28] Arizona law contains the following requirements.

> A. An applicant for licensure as a pharmacy technician must:
> 1. Be of good moral character.
> 2. Be at least eighteen years of age.
> 3. Have a high school diploma or the equivalent of a high school diploma.
> 4. Complete a training program prescribed by board rules.
> 5. Pass a board approved pharmacy technician examination.
> B. An applicant for licensure as a pharmacy technician trainee must:
> 1. Be of good moral character.
> 2. Be at least eighteen years of age.
> 3. Have a high school diploma or the equivalent of a high school diploma.

A number of state laws require pharmacy technicians to meet additional requirements, including:

- Completion of a pharmacy technician certification exam
- Criminal background check
- Additional training to perform certain tasks
- Continuing education

Because the requirements for pharmacy technicians vary by state and are subject to change, pharmacy technicians may contact the state Board of Pharmacy for their particular state for the current requirements.

Minimum Age and High School Graduation or Equivalent

Nearly all states place age requirements on the ability to work as a pharmacy technician either through an express minimum age requirement or implicitly through the requirement to have a high school diploma or the equivalent. The majority of states that specify a minimum age require pharmacy technicians to be 18 years of age or older. However, some states allow pharmacy technicians to be under 18 years of age. Arizona, Alaska, Indiana, Louisiana, Massachusetts, Montana, Nebraska, Nevada, New Hampshire, New Jersey, Oregon, Rhode Island, West Virginia, and Wyoming require that pharmacy technicians be at least 18 years of age. Alabama and Maryland allow pharmacy technicians to be 17 years of age.

Missouri pharmacy law requires pharmacy technicians applying for registration to be at least the minimum legal working age. The Missouri law states:[29]

Any person desiring to assist a pharmacist in the practice of pharmacy as defined in this chapter shall apply to the board of pharmacy for registration as a pharmacy technician. Such applicant shall be, at a minimum, legal working age and shall forward to the board the appropriate fee and written application on a form provided by the board. Such registration shall be the sole authorization permitted to allow persons to assist licensed pharmacists in the practice of pharmacy as defined in this chapter.

Several states, Kentucky, Illinois, and Minnesota, allow a lower age for pharmacy technicians of at least 16 years of age. As an example, the Illinois law for pharmacy technician registration (225 Illinois Statute 85/9) states:

Any person shall be entitled to registration as a registered pharmacy technician who is of the age of 16 or over, has not engaged in conduct or behavior determined to be grounds for discipline under this Act, is of temperate habits, is attending or has graduated from an accredited high school or comparable school or educational institution, and has filed a written application for registration on a form to be prescribed and furnished by the Department for that purpose. The Department shall issue a certificate of registration as a registered pharmacy technician to any applicant who has qualified as aforesaid, and such registration shall be the sole authority required to assist licensed pharmacists in the practice of pharmacy, under the personal supervision of a licensed pharmacist.

Some states such as Massachusetts allow pharmacy technician trainees to be 16 years of age. For example, Massachusetts regulations[30] state:

(1) A pharmacy technician trainee must meet the following requirements:
    (a) be at least 16 years of age;
    (b) be a high school graduate or the equivalent or currently enrolled in a program which awards such degree;
    (c) be of good moral character; and
    (d) not been convicted of a drug related felony or admitted to sufficient facts to warrant such findings.

Because the minimum age and other requirements vary by state and are subject to change, the state Boards of Pharmacy are a resource for the current requirements.

Education, Training, and Certification

Many states require pharmacy technicians to meet education and training requirements as a condition of obtaining a license, registration, permit, or certificate to work as a pharmacy technician. The state laws and regulations define the specific types of education and training programs that are permitted or required. The requirements under state laws and regulations vary considerably. The education and training requirements include programs provided by pharmacy employers, training by the pharmacist-in-charge or pharmacist manager, Board of Pharmacy approved training courses, pharmacy work experience training hours, or pharmacy training through technical programs or accredited training programs (e.g., programs accredited by the American Society for Health-System Pharmacists).

Many states allow pharmacy employer–provided training programs. Many pharmacy employers have extensive training programs for their pharmacy technicians. Some states require pharmacy employer training programs to be approved by the Board of Pharmacy. A number of states require pharmacy technicians to pass an examination, including an examination provided by their pharmacy employer. Some states require that the examination be approved by the Board of Pharmacy. Examples of states requiring pharmacy technicians to pass an examination include Kansas, Indiana, Maryland, Massachusetts, and Virginia. Some states have added training or examination requirements to allow for a higher pharmacist-to-technician ratio. Because of the wide variability and added requirements under certain circumstances, pharmacy technicians are advised to contact the Board of Pharmacy of the state where they are practicing as a technician.

Examples of some state requirements include the following:

▶ California[31] allows pharmacy technicians to complete a training program or pharmacy technician certification as an option to meet the licensure requirements; and requires pharmacy technicians to have a high school diploma or a general educational certificate, and to meet one of the following options for pharmacy technician education:
  ◆ An associate's degree in pharmacy technology,
  ◆ A course of training specified by the Board, or
  ◆ Certification by the Pharmacy Technician Certification Board (PTCB)
▶ Connecticut[32] requires pharmacy technicians to complete initial training as determined by the pharmacist manager with the training prior to performing tasks. The training must include, but not be limited to, on-the-job and related education commensurate with the tasks performed. Pharmacy technician certification examinations are not required, but pharmacy technicians that have passed the Pharmacy Technician Certification Board certification examination or a certification examination approved by the Board are qualified to register.

Connecticut allows a pharmacist to supervise three pharmacy technicians if the third pharmacy technician is certified by a pharmacy technician certification program.[33] The pharmacist manager is required to:

+ Provide in-service training to maintain the continued competence.
+ Document the training; the pharmacy technician must sign the training records.

Examples from other states include the following:

▶ Idaho requires pharmacy technicians to be registered and trained according to the written standards of the pharmacy employer.[34]

▶ Indiana allows pharmacy technicians to complete an education and training program approved by the Board or pass a certification examination offered by a nationally recognized certification body approved by the Board.[35]

▶ Kansas requires the pharmacist-in-charge to assure that there is a pharmacy technician training program to meet the requirements for the pharmacy site and meets the regulatory requirements and requires every person registered as a pharmacy technician to pass an examination approved by the Board within 30 days after becoming registered. Kansas allows a ratio of three pharmacy technicians per pharmacist (normally is two pharmacy technicians to one pharmacist) if at least two of the pharmacy technicians are certified by a pharmacy technician certification examination program.[36]

▶ Maryland allows an individual to meet the registration requirements by passing a national pharmacy technician certification examination program or passing an examination approved by the Board and completing a pharmacy technician training program approved by the Board that includes 160 hours of work experience and is not longer than 6 months.[37]

▶ Massachusetts requires pharmacy technicians to successfully complete a Board-approved pharmacy technician training program, including a program accredited by the American Society of Health-System Pharmacists, a program provided by a branch of the United States Armed Services or Public Health Services, a program with a minimum of 240 hours of instruction (including 120 training hours), or other courses approved by the Board. In addition, a pharmacy technician trainee must work a minimum of 500 hours and pass a Board-approved pharmacy technician assessment examination administered by the employer or a Board-approved national technician certification examination. Massachusetts also allows pharmacy technicians that pass a Board-approved pharmacy technician certification exam to perform additional tasks.[38]

Many states allow pharmacy technicians to be trained through pharmacy employer–provided training programs, including training by the pharmacist-in-charge. Some of these states include Connecticut, Delaware, Idaho, Indiana, Maine, Maryland, North Dakota, Oklahoma, Vermont, and West Virginia. For example, Indiana permits pharmacy technicians to complete an employer training program along with other options, including:[39]

▶ A Board-approved comprehensive education and training program conducted by a pharmacy or an educational organization.
▶ A pharmacy employer technician training program that includes specific training components on technician tasks and duties; patient confidentiality and ethics; pharmacy and medical terminology; abbreviations; symbols commonly used in prescriptions and drug orders; drug storage, packaging, and labeling; pharmacy calculations; drug purchasing and inventory control; and pharmacy record keeping.

Because requirements vary by state and state laws and regulations may change, the state Board of Pharmacy is a resource for the state-specific requirements.

Pharmacy Technician-to-Pharmacist Ratios

Many states have laws and regulations that set a limit on the number of pharmacy technicians that may assist a pharmacist in the pharmacy. These are known as pharmacy technician-to-pharmacist ratios or pharmacy technician ratios. These ratios determine the maximum number of pharmacy technicians that may assist a pharmacist at a given time. For example, if the ratio is three to one (e.g., 3:1) the pharmacist may supervise up to three pharmacy technicians. Generally, pharmacy technician ratios vary from two to one (i.e., 2:1) to four to one (i.e., 4:1); a number of states have no ratio (**Table 6-1**).

Some states allow a higher pharmacy technician ratio if one or more of the pharmacy technicians meets additional requirements such as certification or pursuant to a utilization plan submitted by the pharmacy and approved by the Board of Pharmacy. As with other requirements, the state Boards of Pharmacy are a resource for information on the pharmacy technician ratio in a state.

Certification Examinations

Pharmacy technician certification examinations test proficiency and comprehension of specific areas related to practice as a pharmacy technician. Certification examination programs are offered by private entities, not by state Boards of Pharmacy. Two national pharmacy technician certification examinations exist.[40] State pharmacy laws and regulations have different application certification examinations. Some states allow certification examinations as an option, and others may require pharmacy technicians to pass a certification examination. Some states limit pharmacy technicians to a specific certification examination. Pharmacy technicians may con-

Table 6-1
Pharmacy Technician-to-Pharmacist Ratios

Ratio	States
None	Alaska, Arizona, Delaware, Washington DC, Hawaii, Illinois, Iowa, Kentucky, Maryland, Michigan, Minnesota, Missouri, New Hampshire, Ohio, Oregon, Pennsylvania, Rhode Island, Vermont
1:1	California (1:1 for first pharmacist and 2:1 for additional pharmacist)
2:1	Arkansas, Kansas, Massachusetts (may be 4:1 if third is certified and fourth is a pharmacy intern), Mississippi, Nebraska, Nevada, New Jersey (may be exceeded with plan and certified technicians), New York, North Carolina (may be exceeded if technician certified), Oklahoma, South Carolina (3:1 if second and third technicians certified), South Dakota (4:1 for mail service pharmacies), Tennessee, Texas
3:1	Alabama, Colorado (third technician must be certified, completed accredited program, or completed 500 hours), Connecticut (third technician must be certified), Florida (up to 3:1 with Board approval), Georgia (if third technician certified, passed employer program or certified by PTCB), Idaho, Louisiana (if no technicians are registration candidates; if yes, ratio is 2:1), Maine (if no technicians are "advanced"), Montana (Board may approve higher ratio), Nevada (hospitals), North Dakota, Texas (if no more than two trainees), Utah, Washington (higher with Board approval), Wyoming
4:1	Indiana, Maine (if at least one technician is an "advanced" technician), Massachusetts (if the third and fourth technicians are certified and fourth is an intern pharmacist; otherwise 2:1), New Mexico (Board may allow increase), North Dakota (hospital, closed door, and remote telepharmacies), Virginia, West Virginia, Wisconsin (Board may approve higher ratio with plan)

tact the state Board of Pharmacy with questions regarding the requirements or use of pharmacy technician certification examinations in their state.

In some states, passing a nationally recognized pharmacy technician certification examination is one of the options to meet the criteria for licensure or registration (e.g., California, Connecticut, and Maryland). For example, Connecticut pharmacy law on registration of pharmacy technicians[41] states:

(a) No person shall act as a pharmacy technician unless registered with or certified with, the department.

(b) The department shall, upon authorization of the commission, register as a pharmacy technician any person who presents evidence satisfactory to the department that such person is qualified to perform, under the direct supervision of a pharmacist, routine functions in the dispensing of drugs that do not require the use of professional judgment. The qualifications for registration as a pharmacy technician under this section shall be in accordance with (1) the standards of an institutional pharmacy, a care-giving institution or a correctional or juvenile training institution, in the case of employment in any such pharmacy or institution, or (2) the standards established by regulation adopted by the commissioner in accordance with chapter 54, in the case of employment in a pharmacy. As used in this subsection, "direct supervision" means a supervising pharmacist (A) is physically present in the area or location where the pharmacy is performing routine drug dispensing functions, and (B) conducts in-process and final checks on the pharmacy technician's performance.

(c) *The department shall, upon authorization of the commission, certify as a pharmacy technician any person who meets the requirements for registration as a pharmacy technician, pursuant to subsection (b) of this section, and who holds a certification from the Pharmacy Technician Certification Board or any other equivalent pharmacy technician certification program approved by the department.*

Some states allow pharmacy technicians that pass a certification examination to perform additional duties (e.g., Kentucky, Massachusetts, South Carolina, and Tennessee). For example, Kentucky recognizes pharmacy technicians as certified if they pass the Pharmacy Technician Certification Board examination or the Nuclear Pharmacy Technician Training Program at the University of Tennessee, and allow certified pharmacy technicians to perform certain functions. Kentucky regulations[42] state:

1. A person shall be recognized by the board as a certified pharmacy technician, if:
   (1) (a) He has successfully completed the National Certification Examination administered by the Pharmacy Technician Certification Board; and (b) The certificate issued by the Pharmacy Technician Certification Board is current; or
   (2) He has successfully completed the Nuclear Pharmacy Technician Training Program at the University of Tennessee.
2. A certified pharmacy technician, subject to the supervision, as defined by KRS 315.010(25), of a pharmacist may perform the following functions:
   (1) Certify for delivery unit dose mobile transport systems that have been refilled by another technician;
   (2) Within a nuclear pharmacy, receive diagnostic orders; and
   (3) (a) Initiate or receive a telephonic communication from a practitioner or practitioner's agent concerning refill authorization, after he clearly identifies himself as a certified pharmacy technician; (b) If a practitioner or

practitioner's agent communicates information that does not relate to the refill authorization:

1. A technician shall immediately inform the pharmacist; and
2. The pharmacist shall receive the communication.
3. (1) A technician who has not been certified by the Pharmacy Technician Certification Board may perform the functions specified by Section 2 of this administrative regulation under the immediate supervision of a pharmacist.

   (2) A function performed by a certified pharmacy technician or pharmacy technician shall be performed subject to the review of the pharmacist who directed the technician to perform the function.

   (3) A pharmacist who directs a certified pharmacy technician or pharmacy technician to perform a function shall be responsible for the technician and the performance of the function.

In other states, passing a pharmacy technician certification examination allows the person to be exempt from continuing education requirements (e.g., Alaska, Texas). Texas also requires certification as an initial requirement for licensure.

In a few states, all pharmacy technicians are required (or will be required at a future date) to pass a certification examination in addition to meeting the other training and education requirements. Montana, Rhode Island, Texas (for initial registration), Utah, and Wyoming require all pharmacy technicians to be certified through a pharmacy certification examination. Iowa will require all new pharmacy technicians to pass a national certification examination beginning in July 2010. Oregon will require all pharmacy technicians to pass a certification examination by October 2008, 1 year after initial licensure, or prior to the technician's nineteenth birthday.

Some states allow pharmacies to have a higher pharmacy technician-to-pharmacist ratio if one or more of the pharmacy technicians have passed a pharmacy technician certification exam (e.g., Arizona, Colorado, North Carolina, and Tennessee). Colorado pharmacy law[43] provides an example of a state that requires at least one of three pharmacy technicians on duty to be certified by a national pharmacy technician certification program, or meet other requirements. Colorado law states:

> A pharmacist may supervise up to three persons who are either pharmacy interns or pharmacy technicians, of whom no more than two may be pharmacy interns. *If three pharmacy technicians are on duty, at least one shall be certified by a nationally recognized certification board, possess a degree from an accredited pharmacy technician training program, or have com-*

pleted five hundred hours of experiential training in duties described in section 12-22-102 (26) (b) at the pharmacy as certified by the pharmacist manager. Documentation verifying the training shall be retained within the pharmacy for review by the pharmacist responsible for the final check on prescriptions filled by the pharmacy technician and available for inspection by the board. This supervision ratio does not include other ancillary personnel that may be in the prescription drug outlet, but are not performing duties described in section 12-22-102 (26) (b) that are delegated to such interns or pharmacy technicians.

Some states require that one of the on-duty pharmacy technicians be certified. For example, Alabama pharmacy regulations[44] state:

It is ruled by the Board of Pharmacy that three (3) technicians, one of which shall be certified through the Pharmacy Technician Certification Board (PTCB), on duty are sufficient in the prescription area of a retail pharmacy or an institutional pharmacy for each full time licensed pharmacist on duty. Nothing in this rule shall prevent a pharmacy from employing technicians to perform supervised tasks not requiring professional judgment.

State laws and regulations establishing requirements for education, training, and certification may change. Pharmacy technicians should contact their respective state Board of Pharmacy for complete information on the requirements.

Permitted Acts and Responsibilities

Pharmacy technicians are an important and necessary part of the delivery of pharmacy services, and their assistance allows pharmacists to enhance their provision of pharmacy patient care services. Pharmacy laws and regulations distinguish between the tasks and responsibilities that are restricted to licensed pharmacists and those tasks that pharmacy technicians are permitted to perform as they assist pharmacists. In general, state pharmacy laws and regulations limit pharmacy technicians to performing non-judgmental and nondiscretionary tasks that do not require the professional judgment, education, and training of a pharmacist. State laws and regulations use different language to describe these limits and define the scope of the tasks that pharmacy technicians are allowed to perform.

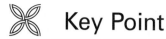 **Key Point**

> Generally, state pharmacy laws and regulations limit pharmacy techni-
> cians to performing tasks that do not require the professional judg-
> ment, education, and training of a pharmacist.

To assist with understanding of how states regulate the permitted tasks that pharmacy technicians may perform, examples of language from several states are provided. Some states define the categories of tasks that pharmacy technicians may perform and state that pharmacy technicians may not perform tasks restricted to the pharmacist. California provides an example of this type of language. California defines the tasks that pharmacy technicians may perform as non-discretionary tasks under the direct supervision and control of a pharmacist *and* specifically states that pharmacy technicians are not permitted to perform any tasks that require the professional judgment of a pharmacist. California law[45] states:

(a) A pharmacy technician may perform packaging, manipulative, repetitive, or other nondiscretionary tasks, only while assisting, and while under the direct supervision and control of a pharmacist.
(b) This section does not authorize the performance of any tasks specified in subdivision (a) by a pharmacy technician without a pharmacist on duty.
(c) This section does not authorize a pharmacy technician to perform any act requiring the exercise of professional judgment by a pharmacist.

California regulations[46] define pharmacy technician in terms of being permitted to perform nondiscretionary tasks, but not performing tasks restricted to a pharmacist.

> Pharmacy technician means an individual who, under the direct su-
> pervision and control of a pharmacist, performs packaging, manipula-
> tive, repetitive, or other nondiscretionary tasks related to the process-
> ing of a prescription in a pharmacy, but who does not perform duties
> restricted to a pharmacist under 1793.1.

Other states define the tasks that pharmacy technicians are not permitted to perform. For instance, Iowa regulations establish the tasks that pharmacy technicians may not perform.[47]

> A pharmacy technician shall not:
> 1. Provide the final verification for the accuracy, validity, completeness,
>   or appropriateness of a filled prescription or medication order;

2. Conduct prospective drug use review or evaluate a patient's medication record for purposes identified in rule 657-8.21(155A);
3. Provide patient counseling, consultation, or patient-specific drug information;
4. Make decisions that require a pharmacist's professional judgment such as interpreting or applying information.

Some states provide a list of the tasks that pharmacy technicians are permitted to perform. Virginia law, for instance, states:[48]

No person shall perform the duties of a pharmacy technician without first being registered as a pharmacy technician with the Board. Upon being registered with the Board as a pharmacy technician, the following tasks may be performed:

1. The entry of prescription information and drug history into a data system or other record keeping system;
2. The preparation of prescription labels or patient information;
3. The removal of the drug to be dispensed from inventory;
4. The counting, measuring, or compounding of the drug to be dispensed;
5. The packaging and labeling of the drug to be dispensed and the repackaging thereof;
6. The stocking or loading of automated dispensing devices or other devices used in the dispensing process;
7. The acceptance of refill authorization from a prescriber or his authorized agency, so long as there is no change to the original prescription; and
8. The performance of any other task restricted to pharmacy technicians by the Board's regulations.

Other states specify that pharmacy technicians may perform only tasks that they are trained and proficient to perform. Rhode Island is an example of a state where the regulations classify pharmacy technicians into two categories, Pharmacy Technician I and Pharmacy Technician II. Pharmacy Technician IIs may perform the task permitted for Pharmacy Technician Is plus additional tasks. Pharmacy Technician Is may perform the following tasks:

23.14 Pharmacy technicians I may perform only those tasks for which they have been trained and in which there is proficiency as determined by the pharmacist-in-charge, but in no case, shall ever exceed what is permitted by regulation, law or scope of practice, and as set forth below:

23.14.1 A pharmacy technician I may request refill authorizations for patients from a prescriber who uses a voice mail response system and/ or when an agent of the prescriber transcribes the requested information for a follow-up phone call to the pharmacy after reviewing the request with the prescriber. The pharmacy technician I may accept authorization for refills from the prescriber or prescriber's agent provided that no information has changed from the previous prescription. 23.14.2 A pharmacy technician I may not perform drug utilization review; clinical conflict resolution, prescriber contact concerning prescription drug order clarification or therapy modification; patient counseling or dispensing process validation; or receive new prescription drug orders or conduct prescription transfers.

Pharmacy Technician IIs are allowed to perform the following additional tasks:

23.15 Pharmacy technician IIs may perform only those tasks for which they have been trained and in which there is proficiency as determined by the pharmacist-in-charge, but in no case, shall ever exceed what is permitted by regulation, law, or scope of practice. In addition to performing the duties and responsibilities stipulated above for pharmacy technician I, pharmacy technicians IIs may perform the following duties:
23.15.1 A pharmacy technician II may request refill authorizations from the prescriber or prescriber's agent and, with the approval of the pharmacist on duty, receive new prescription information and changes to prescriptions from the prescriber or agent, except where otherwise prohibited by federal or state laws and regulations.[49]

The state Boards of Pharmacy are resources for pharmacy technicians to become familiar with the tasks that they are permitted to perform under the state laws and regulations. The state laws and regulations discussed above are examples of how states regulate pharmacy technicians' permitted tasks and functions. Because pharmacy technicians work under the control and supervision of pharmacists, they should consult with their pharmacy employer and supervising pharmacist's direction and become familiar with the laws and regulations of the state where they work as a pharmacy technician.

Quality Improvement Programs

A number of states have enacted laws and regulations that require pharmacies to engage in efforts or quality improvement programs to take steps to prevent mistakes in dispensing prescriptions (also known as misfiling prescriptions). States use different terms in their laws and regulations for these programs such as quality improvement programs, quality assurance programs, or set other requirements for pharmacies to take steps to prevent pharmacy errors. The requirements for these programs vary from state to state. Some states require pharmacies to notify the Board of Pharmacy if a pharmacy mistake results in patient suffering and injury or death. In other states when a pharmacy mistake occurs, the pharmacy is required to review the events surrounding the error and to consider practices to prevent errors from occurring in the future. Examples of states with laws that require pharmacies to have quality improvement or quality assurance programs include Arizona, California, Connecticut, Florida, Iowa, Maryland, Massachusetts, North Carolina, Tennessee, Texas, and West Virginia. Other states require pharmacies to have policies, implement controls, or place responsibility on the pharmacist-in-charge to implement policies to monitor and prevent errors (e.g., Kansas, Kentucky, Minnesota, Oklahoma, New Mexico, and Rhode Island). Some states require that misfilled prescriptions be reported to the Board of Pharmacy (e.g., Georgia and New Mexico).

California provides an example of a law requiring pharmacies to establish a quality assurance program to document pharmacy medication errors and take appropriate actions to prevent a recurrence.

> Every pharmacy shall establish a quality assurance program that shall, at a minimum, document medication errors attributable, in whole or in part, to the pharmacy or its personnel. The purpose of the quality assurance program shall be to assess errors that occur in the pharmacy in dispensing or furnishing prescription medications so that the pharmacy may take appropriate action to prevent a recurrence.[50]

The California Board of Pharmacy issued regulations[51] to establish the requirements for pharmacy quality assurance programs. For instance, if the pharmacist becomes aware of an error, the pharmacist is required to notify the patient, take steps to lessen the effect of the error, and notify the patient's prescriber if the patient received the drug. The regulations also require pharmacies to use the findings of the quality assurance program to develop pharmacy systems and processes to prevent medication errors.

(a) Each pharmacy shall establish or participate in an established quality assurance program which documents and assesses medication errors to determine cause and an appropriate response as part of a mission to improve the quality of pharmacy service and prevent errors.

(b) For purposes of this section, "medication error" means any variation from a prescription or drug order not authorized by the prescriber, as described in

Section 1716. Medication error, as defined in the section, does not include any variation that is corrected prior to furnishing the drug to the patient or patient's agent or any variation allowed by law.

(c) (1) Each quality assurance program shall be managed in accordance with written policies and procedures maintained in the pharmacy in an immediately retrievable form.

(2) When a pharmacist determines that a medication error has occurred, a pharmacist shall as soon as possible:

(A) Communicate to the patient or the patient's agent the fact that a medication error has occurred and the steps required to avoid injury or mitigate the error.

(B) Communicate to the prescriber the fact that a medication error has occurred.

(3) The communication requirement in paragraph (2) of this subdivision shall only apply to medication errors if the drug was administered to or by the patient, or if the medication error resulted in a clinically significant delay in therapy.

(4) If a pharmacist is notified of a prescription error by the patient, the patient's agent, or a prescriber, the pharmacist is not required to communicate with that individual as required in paragraph (2) of this subdivision.

(d) Each pharmacy shall use the findings of its quality assurance program to develop pharmacy systems and workflow processes designed to prevent medication errors. An investigation of each medication error shall commence as soon as is reasonably possible, but no later than 2 business days from the date the medication error is discovered. All medication errors discovered shall be subject to a quality assurance review.

(e) The primary purpose of the quality assurance review shall be to advance error prevention by analyzing, individually and collectively, investigative and other pertinent data collected in response to a medication error to assess the cause and any contributing factors such as system or process failures. A record of the quality assurance review shall be immediately retrievable in the pharmacy. The record shall contain at least the following:

(1) the date, location, and participants in the quality assurance review;

(2) the pertinent data and other information relating to the medication error(s) reviewed and documentation of any patient contact required by subdivision (c);

(3) the findings and determinations generated by the quality assurance review; and,

(4) recommend changes to pharmacy policy, procedure, systems, or processes, if any.

The pharmacy shall inform pharmacy personnel of changes to pharmacy policy, procedure, systems, or processes made as a result of recommendations generated in the quality assurance program.

Kansas is an example of a state requiring the pharmacist-in-charge to develop policies and procedures to document prescription dispensing errors. Kansas regulations[52] set the following requirements for pharmacy errors.

Incident reports

(a) For each pharmacy other than a medical care pharmacy, the pharmacist-in-charge shall ensure that procedures exist requiring each pharmacist who becomes aware of an alleged or real error in filling or dispensing a prescription to report the incident to the pharmacist-in-charge as soon as practical.

(b) As soon as possible after discovery of the incident, the pharmacist shall prepare a report containing the following information:

(1) the name, address, age, and phone number of any complainant, if available;

(2) the name of each pharmacy employee and the license number of each licensee involved;

(3) the date of the incident and the date of the report;

(4) a description of the incident;

(5) the prescriber's name and whether or not the prescriber was contacted;

(6) a description of the actions taken as a result of the incident;

(7) the steps taken to prevent a recurrence; and

(8) the signatures of all pharmacy employees involved in the incident.
    For each pharmacy, the pharmacist-in-charge shall ensure that procedures exist requiring that the incident report be maintained in the pharmacy for at least five years in a manner so that the report can be provided to the board or its representative immediately upon request.

(c) The preparation of an incident report that meets the requirements of this regulation shall be the responsibility of each pharmacist involved in the incident and the pharmacist-in-charge. The maintenance of incident reports as required by this regulation shall be the responsibility of the pharmacist-in-charge.

Pharmacy technicians have an important role in assuring the correct dispensing of prescription drugs by carefully undertaking and completing their duties and responsibilities. Pharmacy technicians should also immediately notify the pharmacist on duty if they become aware of a pharmacy error or if they are contacted by a patient with any questions or concerns about their prescription medications.

Patient Counseling

Patient counseling by pharmacists is covered in state and federal regulation. As discussed in Chapter 3, pharmacist patient counseling is addressed federally in the Omnibus Budget Reconciliation Act of 1990 (OBRA '90). OBRA '90 established a requirement for pharmacists to offer to counsel state Medicaid patients regarding their prescriptions. Pharmacists are required to offer to counsel patients on how to take the drug, the dosage, how long to take the drug, common side effects, how to avoid contraindications, drugs or foods that should not be taken with their medication, proper drug storage, what to do if a dose is missed, and information on refilling their medication.

In addition to OBRA '90, state pharmacy laws and regulations set requirements for pharmacist counseling of patients regarding their prescription medications. The state requirements for patient counseling vary from state to state with some states having stronger requirements than OBRA '90. For example, most states require that the offer to counsel be provided to all patients, not just Medicaid patients. Some of the other differences among the states include whether an offer to counsel is required on new prescriptions or both new and refill prescriptions, whether counseling is mandatory, whether pharmacists may use professional judgment on when to provide counseling, whether the offer to counsel must be made by the pharmacist or may be made by a nonpharmacist, whether a pharmacy intern may provide the counseling under the pharmacist's supervision, whether the counseling may be provided by other than oral means such as written counseling materials and by telephone, and whether counseling or the patient's or the caregiver's refusal of counseling must be documented. The state laws and regulations for patient counseling are diverse.

State pharmacy patient counseling laws and regulations address who is permitted to make the offer to counsel, including whether the offer to counsel must be made by the pharmacist or whether a nonpharmacist may make the offer to counsel. State requirements also vary on whether an offer to counsel is required on refill prescriptions. For example, some states require an offer to counsel on refilled prescriptions if the refilled prescription has a different strength, dosage form, or directions for use. Other states require an offer to counsel yearly on refill prescriptions for maintenance medications. Some states require an offer to counsel on refilled prescriptions based on the pharmacist's professional judgment.

An important distinction for pharmacy technicians is the difference between the "offer to counsel" and providing counseling to the patient or the patient's caregiver. All states require that the patient counseling be provided by the pharmacist. Some states allow pharmacy interns to provide counseling under the pharmacist's supervision. Pharmacy technicians are not authorized to provide patient counseling.

Pharmacy technicians should be familiar with the requirement in their state for who may make the offer to counsel. The state Boards of Pharmacy are a resource for further information on the specific requirements in each state.

Summary

State pharmacy laws and regulations set requirements for pharmacy practice such as licensure of pharmacies and pharmacists, scope of pharmacy practice for pharmacists, and pharmacist-in-charge requirements. Many states have laws and regulations regulating pharmacy technicians, including registration or licensure, tasks that pharmacy technicians may perform, and responsibilities that may only be performed by pharmacists. Each state has its own pharmacy laws and regulations with specific requirements varying by state, including the requirements applicable to a pharmacy technicians.

State Boards of Pharmacy are the primary state agency responsible for oversight, discipline, and rulemaking authority for pharmacy practice, including rules and regulations covering pharmacy technicians. Common regulatory requirements for pharmacy technicians include registration or licensure, minimum age, training and education, examinations, certification examinations, criminal background checks, technician-to-pharmacist ratios, permitted duties, prohibited conduct, and disciplinary penalties.

References

1. Iowa Code 155A.3.
2. Iowa Code 155A.13.
3. California Business and Professions Code Section 4037.
4. California Business and Professions Code Section 4117.
5. California Business and Professions Code Section 4343.
6. Wisconsin Act, 2005. Act 242. Wisconsin Statutes 450.065.
7. Oregon Revised Statutes 689.315.
8. Iowa Code 155A.8.
9. Knapp et al. Update on the Pharmacist Shortage: National and State Data through 2003. *Am J Health-Syst Pharm*. 2005:62(5):492-9.
10. California Business and Professions Code Section 4001.5.
11. Oregon Revised Statutes 689.356.
12. New Jersey Statutes 45:14-48(b).
13. New Mexico Statutes 61-11-6.
14. California Business and Professions Code Section 4301
15. California Business and Professions Code Section 4306.5.
16. Alaska statutes 08.80.030 (b)(9).
17. Arizona Statutes 32-1923.01.
18. California Business and Professions Code Section 4115(e).
19. Oregon Revised Statutes Section 689.151.
20. Rhode Island Statutes 5-19.1-5.
21. Utah Statutes 58-17b-301.

22. Wyoming Statutes 1977 Section 33-24-301.
23. Minnesota Statutes Section 151.06.
24. Montana Code Section 37-7-201.
25. New Jersey Statutes 45:14-48.
26. 59 Oklahoma Statutes Section 353.29(B).
27. West Virginia Code Section 30-5-5a.
28. Arizona Statutes 32-1923.01.
29. Missouri Statutes 338.013.
30. Massachusetts Code of Regulations 8.03.
31. California Business and Professions Code Section 4202.
32. Connecticut Regulations 20-576-37.
33. Connecticut General Statutes Section 50-598a.
34. Idaho Administrative Code 27.01.01.251.
35. Indiana Code 25-26-19-5.
36. Kansas Statutes 65-1663; Kansas regulations 68-5-15.
37. Maryland Statutes 12-6B-02.
38. Code of Massachusetts Regulations Section 8.02 and 8.04.
39. Indiana Administrative Code 856 IAC 1-35-4.
40. Pharmacy Technician Certification Board (PTCB), see www.ptcb.org; and Institute for Certification of Pharmacy Technicians (ICPT), see www.nationaltechexam.org.
41. Connecticut General Statutes 20-598a.
42. Kentucky Regulations 201 KAR 2:045.
43. Colorado Statutes 12-22-121.7.
44. Alabama Regulations 680-X-2-.14.
45. California Business and Professions Code Section 4115.
46. California Administrative Code Title 16, Section 1793.
47. Iowa Administrative Code 657-3.23(155A).
48. Virginia Code Section 54.1-3321:045.
49. Rhode Island Regulations Part V, Section 23.
50. California Business and Professions Code Section 4125.
51. California Pharmacy regulation Section 1711.
52. Kansas Regulations 68-7-12b.

Self-Assessment Questions

1. What state agency has the authority, oversight, and enforcement power over the licensure and registration of pharmacy technicians with the state?
2. In addition to licensure and/or registration, what are three other possible requirements a state may demand of pharmacy technicians?
3. Define "pharmacy technician ratios."
4. What types of tasks are pharmacy technicians limited to performing in the pharmacy?
5. What is the PTCB?

Appendix 6-1. NABP MODEL ACT Article IV—Discipline

Introductory Comment to Article IV

At the very heart of any Pharmacy Act is the enforcement power of the Board of Pharmacy. The Board must have authority to discipline and/or prohibit Pharmacists, Pharmacy Interns, Certified Pharmacy Technicians, or Pharmacy Technicians who violate this Act or Rules from continuing to threaten the public if it is to fulfill its responsibilities. The Board must have the ability to stop wrongdoers, either permanently or temporarily, discipline them, and, where appropriate, to guide and assist errant licensees in rehabilitating themselves. The Model Act *disciplinary provisions are contained in Article IV. They were drafted with the purpose of granting to the Board the widest possible scope within which to perform its disciplinary functions. Standardized disciplinary action terms and definitions were developed to facilitate the accurate reporting of disciplinary actions taken by Boards of Pharmacy and to avoid confusion associated with state-to-state variations in terms and definitions. The grounds for disciplinary action were developed to ensure protection of the public, while reserving to the Board the power to expand upon them and adapt them to changing or local conditions as necessary. The penalties permitted under the* Model Act *will afford the Board the flexibility to conform and relate discipline to offenses.*

Section 401. Disciplinary Action Terms

The following is a list of disciplinary actions which may be taken, issued, or assessed by the Board of Pharmacy: Revocation, Summary Suspension, Suspension, Probation, Censure, Reprimand, Warning, Cease and Desist, Fine/Civil Penalty, Costs/Administrative Costs.

Section 402. Grounds, Penalties, and Reinstatement

(a) The Board of Pharmacy may refuse to issue or renew, or may Revoke, Summarily Suspend, Suspend, place on Probation, Censure, Reprimand, issue a Warning against, or issue a Cease and Desist order against, the licenses or the registration of, or assess a Fine/Civil Penalty or Costs/Administrative Costs against any Person Pursuant to the procedures set forth in Section 403 herein below, upon one or more of the following grounds:

(1) Unprofessional conduct as that term is defined by the rules of the Board;

(2) Incapacity that prevents a licensee from engaging in the Practice of Pharmacy or a registrant from assisting in the Practice of Pharmacy, with reasonable skill, competence, and safety to the public;

(3) Being guilty of one (1) or more of the following:
   (i) a felony;
   (ii) any act involving moral turpitude or gross immorality; or
   (iii) violations of the Pharmacy or Drug laws of this State or rules and regulations pertaining thereto; or of laws, rules, and regulations of any other state; or of the Federal government;

(4) Disciplinary action taken by another state or jurisdiction against a license or other authorization to Practice Pharmacy based upon conduct by the licensee similar to conduct that would constitute grounds for actions as defined in this section;

(5) Failure to report to the Board any adverse action taken by another licensing jurisdiction (United States or foreign), government agency, law enforcement agency, or court for conduct that would constitute grounds for action as defined in this section;

(6) Failure to report to the Board one's surrender of a license or authorization to Practice Pharmacy in another state or jurisdiction while under disciplinary investigation by any of those authorities or bodies for conduct that would constitute grounds for action as defined in this section;

(7) Failure to report to the Board any adverse judgment, settlement, or award arising from a malpractice claim arising related to conduct that would constitute grounds for action as defined in this section;

(8) Knowing or suspecting that a Pharmacist or Pharmacy Intern is incapable of engaging in the Practice of Pharmacy or that a Pharmacy Technician is incapable of assisting in the Practice of Pharmacy, with reasonable skill, competence, and safety to the public, and failing to report any relevant information to the Board of Pharmacy;

(9) Misrepresentation of a material fact by a licensee in securing the issuance or renewal of a license or registration;

(10) Fraud by a licensee in connection with the Practice of Pharmacy;

(11) Engaging, or aiding and abetting an individual to engage in the Practice of Pharmacy without a license; assisting in the Practice of Pharmacy or aiding and abetting an individual to assist in the Practice of Pharmacy without having registered with the Board of Pharmacy; or falsely using the title of Pharmacist, Pharmacy Intern, Certified Pharmacy Technician, or Pharmacy Technician;

(12) Failing to pay the costs assessed in a disciplinary hearing pursuant to Section 213(b)(9);

(13) Engaging in any conduct that subverts or attempts to subvert any licensing examination or the administration of any licensing examination;

(14) Being found by the Board to be in violation of any of the provisions of this Act or rules adopted pursuant to this Act;

(15) Illegal use or disclosure of Protected Health Information;

(16) Failure to furnish to the Board, its investigators, or representatives any information legally requested by the Board.

   (b)   (1)   The Board may defer action with regard to an impaired licensee who voluntarily signs an agreement, in a form satisfactory to the Board, agreeing not to practice Pharmacy and to enter an approved treatment and monitoring program in accordance with this Section, provided that this Section should not apply to a licensee who has been convicted of, pleads guilty to, or enters a plea of nolo contendere to a felonious act prohibited by or a conviction relating to a controlled substance in a court of law of the United States or any other state, territory, or country. A licensee who is physically or mentally impaired due to addiction to Drugs or alcohol may qualify as an impaired Pharmacist and have disciplinary action deferred and ultimately waived only if the Board is satisfied that such action will not endanger the public and the licensee enters into an agreement with the Board for a treatment and monitoring plan approved by the Board, progresses satisfactorily in such treatment and monitoring program, complies with all terms of the agreement and all other applicable terms of subsection (2)(b). Failure to enter such agreement or to comply with the terms and make satisfactory progress in the treatment and monitoring program shall disqualify the licensee from the provisions of this Section and the Board shall activate an immediate investigation and disciplinary proceedings. Upon completion of the rehabilitation program in accordance with the agreement signed by the Board, the licensee may apply for permission to resume the Practice of Pharmacy upon such conditions as the Board determines necessary.

(2)   The Board may require a licensee to enter into an agreement which includes, but is not limited to, the following provisions:

    (i)   Licensee agrees that his or her license shall be Suspended or Revoked indefinitely under subsection (b)(1).

    (ii)   Licensee will enroll in a treatment and monitoring program approved by the Board.

    (iii)   Licensee agrees that failure to satisfactorily progress in such treatment and monitoring program shall be reported to the Board by the treating professional, who shall be immune from any liability for such reporting made in good faith.

    (iv)   Licensee consents to the treating physician or professional of the approved treatment and monitoring program reporting to the Board on the progress of licensee at such intervals as the Board deems necessary and such Person making such report will not be liable when such reports are made in good faith.

(3)   The ability of an impaired Pharmacist to practice shall only be restored and charges dismissed when the Board is satisfied by the reports it has received from the approved treatment program that licensee can resume practice without danger to the public.

(4)   Licensee consents, in accordance with applicable law, to the release of any treatment information from anyone within the approved treatment program.

(5)   The impaired licensee who has enrolled in an approved treatment and monitoring program and entered into an agreement with the Board in accordance with subsection (b)(1) hereof shall have his license Suspended or Revoked, but enforcement of this Suspension or Revocation shall be stayed by the length of time the licensee remains in the program and makes satisfactorily progress, and complies with the terms of the agreement and adheres to any limitations on his practice imposed by the Board to protect the public. Failure to enter into such agreement or to comply with the terms and make satisfactory progress in the treatment and monitoring program shall disqualify the licensee from the provisions of this Section and the Board

shall activate an immediate investigation and disciplinary proceedings.

(6) Any Pharmacist who has substantial evidence that a licensee has an active addictive disease for which the licensee is not receiving treatment under a program approved by the Board pursuant to an agreement entered into under this Section, is diverting a controlled substance, or is mentally or physically incompetent to carry out the duties of his/her license, shall make or cause to be made a report to the Board. Any Person who reports pursuant to this Section in good faith and without malice shall be immune from any civil or criminal liability arising from such reports. Failure to provide such a report within a reasonable time from receipt of knowledge may be considered grounds for disciplinary action against the licensee so failing to report.

(c) Any Person whose license to practice Pharmacy in this State has been Revoked, Summarily Suspended, Suspended, placed on Probation, Censured, Reprimanded, issued a Warning against, or issued a Cease and Desist order against, the licenses or the registration of, or assessed a Fine/Civil Penalty or Costs/Administrative Costs against pursuant to this Act, whether voluntarily or by action of the Board, shall have the right, at reasonable intervals, to petition the Board for reinstatement of such license. Such petition shall be made in writing and in the form prescribed by the Board. Upon investigation and hearing, the Board may, in its discretion, grant or deny such petition, or it may modify its original finding to reflect any circumstances that have changed sufficiently to warrant such modifications. The Board, also at its discretion, may require such Person to pass an examination(s) for reentry into the Practice of Pharmacy.

(d) Nothing herein shall be construed as barring criminal prosecutions for violations of this Act.

(e) All final decisions by the Board shall be subject to judicial review pursuant to the Administrative Procedures Act.

(f) Any individual or entity whose license to practice Pharmacy, or registration to assist in the Practice of Pharmacy, is Revoked, Suspended, or not renewed shall return his or her license or registration certificate to the offices of the State Board of Pharmacy within ten days after receipt of notice of such action.

Section 403. Procedure

(a) Notwithstanding any provisions of the State Administrative Procedures Act, the Board may, without a hearing, Summarily Suspend a license for not more than 60 days if the Board finds that a Pharmacist, Pharmacy Intern, Certified Pharmacy Technician, or Pharmacy Technician has violated a law or rule that the Board is empowered to enforce, and if continued practice by the Pharmacist, Pharmacy Intern, Certified Pharmacy Technician, or Pharmacy Technician would create an imminent risk of harm to the public. The Suspension shall take effect upon written notice to the Pharmacist, Pharmacy Intern, Certified Pharmacy Technician, or Pharmacy Technician specifying the statute or rule violated. At the time it issues the Suspension notice, the Board shall schedule a disciplinary hearing to be held under the Administrative Procedures Act within 20 days thereafter. The Pharmacist, Pharmacy Intern, Certified Pharmacy Technician, or Pharmacy Technician shall be provided with at least 10 days notice of any hearing held under this subsection.

(b) Notwithstanding any provisions of the State Administrative Procedures Act, the Board may, in its own name, issue a Cease and Desist order to stop an individual from engaging in an unauthorized Practice of Pharmacy or violating or threatening to violate a statute, rule, or order which the Board has issued or is empowered to enforce. The Cease and Desist order must state the reason for its issuance and give notice of the individual's right to request a hearing under applicable procedures as set forth in the Administrative Procedures Act. Nothing herein shall be construed as barring criminal prosecutions for violations of this Act.

Section 401. Comment

Guidelines for the imposition of sanctions for certain designated offenses can be found in Appendix E: Guidelines for Disciplinary Sanctions of the Model Act.

Section 402. Comment

The penalties provided in Section 402 give the Board wide latitude to make the disciplinary action fit the offense. The "reasonable intervals" in 402(c) would be determined by the Board.

Section 402(a)(1). Comment

It is particularly important to emphasize the need for specificity in defining the grounds upon which a Pharmacist's or Pharmacy Intern's license to practice Pharmacy, or a Certified Pharmacy Technician's or Pharmacy Technician's registration to assist in the Practice of Pharmacy, may be Revoked or Suspended. The term "unprofessional conduct" is particularly susceptible to judicial challenge for being unconstitutionally vague. Each offense included within the meaning of this term must be capable of being understood with reasonable precision by the Persons regulated so that it can be readily enforced and relied upon during disciplinary proceedings, and so that those regulated by it may easily conform their professional conduct to its meaning(s).

These potential problems make it essential for Boards to issue appropriate rules making the grounds for disciplinary action specific, understandable, and reasonable. In addition, the Boards must ensure that such rules are published for the benefit of all licensees within their jurisdiction. Only by doing so can Boards be assured of authority to take successful and meaningful disciplinary actions that will not later be overturned by the courts.

This section must be examined in light of other state laws since some states, for example, restrict the circumstances under which a license may be denied to an individual because of the commission of a felony. In addition, an individual who has been convicted of a felony or an act involving gross immorality and who has paid his debt to society has restored constitutional protections that may curtail a strict application of Section 402(a)(3).

Section 402(a)(13). Comment

It is recommended that the following rule be adopted defining subversion or the attempt to subvert any licensing examination.

(a) Conduct which subverts or attempts to subvert any licensing examination or the administration of any examination shall include, but not be limited to, the following:

    (1) Conduct which violates the security of the examination materials; removing from the examination room any examination materials without authorization; the unauthorized reproduction by any means of any portion of the actual licensing examination; aiding by any means the unauthorized reproduction of any portion of the actual licensing examination; paying or using professional or paid examination takers for the purpose of reconstructing any portion of the licensing examination; obtaining examination questions or other examination materials, except by specific authorization either before, during, or after an examination; or selling, distributing, buying, receiving, or having unauthorized possession of any portion of a future, current, or previously administered licensing examination.

    (2) Unauthorized communication of examination information with any other examinee during the administration of a licensing examination;

copying answers from another examinee or permitting one's answers to be copied by another examinee; having in one's possession during the administration of the licensing examination any books, equipment, notes, written or printed materials, or data of any kind other than the examination materials distributed, or otherwise authorized to be in one's possession during the examination; or impersonating any examinee or having an impersonator take the licensing examination on one's behalf.

Section 402(c). Comment

A Pharmacist who is under investigation or who has been charged with a violation of the Pharmacy Practice Act may agree to voluntarily surrender his or her license. When this occurs, the Board should formally enter stipulated findings and an order describing the terms and conditions of the surrender including any agreed upon time limitations. This establishes statutory grounds that would support disciplinary action, and prevents a Pharmacist who has surrendered a license from applying for reinstatement within a time frame unacceptable to the Board.

Section 403. Comment

The procedures which must be followed before disciplinary action can be taken in many of the states are determined by the Administrative Procedures Act. The Model Act was drafted on the assumption that such an Act was in effect.

(Reprinted, with permission, from Model State Pharmacy Act and Model Rules of the National Association of Boards of Pharmacy, August, 2006.)

Appendix 6-2. State Boards of Pharmacy

Alabama State Board of Pharmacy
10 Inverness Center, Suite 110
Birmingham, AL 35242
Phone: 205/981-2280
Fax: 205/981-2330
www.albop.com

Alaska State Board of Pharmacy
PO Box 110806
Juneau, AK 99811-0806
Phone: 907/465-2589
Fax: 907/465-2974
www.commerce.state.ak.us/occ/ppha.htm

Arizona State Board of Pharmacy
4425 W Olive Ave, Suite 140
Glendale, AZ 85302-3844
Phone: 623/463-2727
Fax: 623/934-0583
www.pharmacy.state.az.us

Arkansas State Board of Pharmacy
101 E Capitol, Suite 218
Little Rock, AR 72201
Phone: 501/682-0190
Fax: 501/682-0195
www.arkansas.gov/asbp

California State Board of Pharmacy
1625 N Market Blvd, N219
Sacramento, CA 95834
Phone: 916/574-7900
Fax: 916/574-8618
www.pharmacy.ca.gov/

Colorado State Board of Pharmacy
1560 Broadway, Suite 1310
Denver, CO 80202-5143
Phone: 303/894-7800
Fax: 303/894-7764
www.dora.state.co.us/pharmacy

Connecticut Commission of Pharmacy
State Office Building, 165 Capitol Ave, Room 147
Hartford, CT 06106
Phone: 860/713-6070
Fax: 860/713-7242
www.ct.gov/dcp/site/default.asp

Delaware State Board of Pharmacy
Division of Professional Regulation
Cannon Building
861 Silver Lake Blvd, Suite 203
Dover, DE 19904
Phone: 302/744-4526
Fax: 302/739-2711

District of Columbia Board of Pharmacy
717 14th St NW, Suite 600
Washington, DC 20005
Phone: 202/724-4900
Fax: 202/727-8471
www.dchealth.dc.gov

Florida State Board of Pharmacy
4052 Bald Cypress Way, Bin #C04
Tallahassee, FL 32399-3254
Phone: 850/245-4292
Fax: 850/413-6982
www.doh.state.fl.us/mqa

Georgia State Board of Pharmacy

Professional Licensing Boards
237 Coliseum Dr
Macon, GA 31217-3858
Phone: 478/207-1610
Fax: 478/207-1633
www.sos.state.ga.us/plb/pharmacy

Guam Board of Examiners of Pharmacy

PO Box 2816
Hagatna, GU 96932
Phone: 671/735-7406 ext 11
Fax: 671/735-7413

Hawaii State Board of Pharmacy

PO Box 3469
Honolulu, HI 96801
Phone: 808/586-2694
Fax: 808/586-2874
www.hawaii.gov/dcca/areas/pvl/boards/pharmacy

Idaho State Board of Pharmacy

3380 Americana Terrace, Suite 320
Boise, ID 83706
Phone: 208/334-2356
Fax: 208/334-3536
www.accessidaho.org/bop/

Illinois State Board of Pharmacy

320 W Washington, 3rd Floor
Springfield, IL 62786
Phone: 217/782-8556
Fax: 217/782-7645
www.idfpr.com

Indiana State Board of Pharmacy

402 W Washington St, Room W072
Indianapolis, IN 46204-2739
Phone: 317/234-2067
Fax: 317/233-4236
www.in.gov/pla/bandc/isbp/

Iowa State Board of Pharmacy Examiners
400 SW 8th St, Suite E
Des Moines, IA 50309-4688
Phone: 515/281-5944
Fax: 515/281-4609
www.state.ia.us/ibpe

Kansas State Board of Pharmacy
Landon State Office Building, 900 Jackson, Room 560
Topeka, KS 66612-1231
Phone: 785/296-4056
Fax: 785/296-8420
www.kansas.gov/pharmacy

Kentucky State Board of Pharmacy
Spindletop Administration Bldg, Suite 302
2624 Research Park Dr
Lexington, KY 40511
Phone: 859/246-2820
Fax: 859/246-2823
http://pharmacy.ky.gov/

Louisiana State Board of Pharmacy
5615 Corporate Blvd, Suite 8E
Baton Rouge, LA 70808-2537
Phone: 225/925-6496
Fax: 225/925-6499
www.labp.com

Maine State Board of Pharmacy
Department of Professional/Financial Regulation
35 State House Station
Augusta, ME 04333
Phone: 207/624-8689
Fax: 207/624-8637
www.maineprofessionalreg.org

Maryland State Board of Pharmacy
4201 Patterson Ave
Baltimore, MD 21215-2299
Phone: 410/764-4755
Fax: 410/358-6207
www.dhmh.state.md.us/pharmacyboard/

Massachusetts State Board of Registration in Pharmacy
239 Causeway St, 2nd Floor
Boston, MA 02114
Phone: 617/973-0950
Fax: 617/973-0983
www.mass.gov/dpl/boards/ph/index.htm

Michigan State Board of Pharmacy
611 W Ottawa, First Floor
PO Box 30670
Lansing, MI 48909-8170
Phone: 517/335-0918
Fax: 517/373-2179
www.michigan.gov/healthlicense

Minnesota State Board of Pharmacy
2829 University Ave SE, Suite 530
Minneapolis, MN 55414-3251
Phone: 651/201-2825
Fax: 651/201-2837
www.phcybrd.state.mn.us

Mississippi State Board of Pharmacy
204 Key Dr, Suite D
Madison, MS 39110
Phone: 601/605-5388
Fax: 601/605-9546
www.mbp.state.ms.us

Missouri State Board of Pharmacy

PO Box 625
Jefferson City, MO 65102
Phone: 573/751-0091
Fax: 573/526-3464
www.pr.mo.gov/pharmacists.asp

Montana State Board of Pharmacy

PO Box 200513
301 S Park Ave, 4th Floor
Helena, MT 59620-0513
Phone: 406/841-2371
Fax: 406/841-2305
www.mt.gov/dli/bsd/license/bsd_boards/pha_board/board_page.asp

Nebraska State Board of Pharmacy

PO Box 94986
Lincoln, NE 68509-4986
Phone: 402/471-2118
Fax: 402/471-3577
www.hhs.state.ne.us

Nevada State Board of Pharmacy

555 Double Eagle Ct, Suite 1100
Reno, NV 89521
Phone: 775/850-1440
Fax: 775/850-1444
www.bop.nv.gov

New Hampshire State Board of Pharmacy

57 Regional Dr
Concord, NH 03301-8518
Phone: 603/271-2350
Fax: 603/271-2856
www.nh.gov/pharmacy

New Jersey State Board of Pharmacy
124 Halsey St
Newark, NJ 07101
Phone: 973/504-6450
Fax: 973/648-3355
http://www.state.nj.us/lps/ca/boards.htm

New Mexico State Board of Pharmacy
5200 Oakland NE, Suite A
Albuquerque, NM 87113
Phone: 505/222-9830
Fax: 505/222-9845
www.state.nm.us/pharmacy

New York State Board of Pharmacy
89 Washington Ave, 2nd Floor W
Albany, NY 12234-1000
Phone: 518/474-3817 ext. 130
Fax: 518/473-6995
www.op.nysed.gov

North Carolina State Board of Pharmacy
PO Box 4560
Chapel Hill, NC 27515-4560
Phone: 919/246-1050
Fax: 919/246-1056
www.ncbop.org

North Dakota State Board of Pharmacy
PO Box 1354
Bismarck, ND 58502-1354
Phone: 701/328-9535
Fax: 701/328-9536
www.nodakpharmacy.com

Ohio State Board of Pharmacy
77 S High St, Room 1702
Columbus, OH 43215-6126
Phone: 614/466-4143
Fax: 614/752-4836
www.pharmacy.ohio.gov

Oklahoma State Board of Pharmacy

4545 Lincoln Blvd, Suite 112
Oklahoma City, OK 73105-3488
Phone: 405/521-3815
Fax: 405/521-3758
www.pharmacy.ok.gov

Oregon State Board of Pharmacy

800 NE Oregon St, Suite 150
Portland, OR 97232
Phone: 971/673-0001
Fax: 971/673-0002
www.pharmacy.state.or.us

Pennsylvania State Board of Pharmacy

PO Box 2649
Harrisburg, PA 17105-2649
Phone: 717/783-7156
Fax: 717/787-7769
www.dos.state.pa.us/pharm

Puerto Rico Board of Pharmacy

Call Box 10200
Santurce, PR 00908
Phone: 787/724-7282
Fax: 787/725-7903

Rhode Island State Board of Pharmacy

3 Capitol Hill, Room 205
Providence, RI 02908-5097
Phone: 401/222-2837
Fax: 401/222-2158
www.health.ri.gov/hsr/professions/pharmacy.php

South Carolina State Board of Pharmacy

Kingstree Bldg
110 Centerview Dr, Suite 306
Columbia, SC 29210
Phone: 803/896-4700
Fax: 803/896-4596
www.llronline.com/POL/pharmacy

South Dakota State Board of Pharmacy
4305 S Louise Ave, Suite 104
Sioux Falls, SD 57106
Phone: 605/362-2737
Fax: 605/362-2738
www.state.sd.us/doh/pharmacy

Tennessee State Board of Pharmacy
Tennessee Department of Commerce and Insurance
Board of Pharmacy
Davy Crockett Tower, 2nd Floor
500 James Robertson Pkwy
Nashville, TN 37243-1149
Phone: 615/741-2718
Fax: 615/741-2722
www.state.tn.us/commerce/boards/pharmacy

Texas State Board of Pharmacy
333 Guadalupe, Tower 3, Suite 600
Austin, TX 78701-3942
Phone: 512/305-8000
Fax: 512/305-8082
www.tsbp.state.tx.us

Utah State Board of Pharmacy
PO Box 146741
Salt Lake City, UT 84114-6741
Phone: 801/530-6179
Fax: 801/530-6511
www.dopl.utah.gov/

Vermont State Board of Pharmacy
Office of Professional Regulation
26 Terrace St
Montpelier, VT 05609-1106
Phone: 802/828-2373
Fax: 802/828-2465
www.vtprofessionals.org

Virgin Island Board of Pharmacy
Department of Health
Roy L. Schneider Hospital
48 Sugar Estate
St Thomas, VI 00802
Phone: 340/774-0117
Fax: 340/777-4001

Virginia State Board of Pharmacy
6603 W Broad St, 5th Floor
Richmond, VA 23230-1712
Phone: 804/662-9911
Fax: 804/662-9313
www.dhp.state.va.us/pharmacy/default.htm

Washington State Board of Pharmacy
PO Box 47863
Olympia, WA 98504-7863
Phone: 360/236-4825
Fax: 360/586-4359
fortress.wa.gov/doh/hpqa1/hps4/pharmacy/default.htm

West Virginia State Board of Pharmacy
232 Capitol St
Charleston, WV 25301
Phone: 304/558-0558
Fax: 304/558-0572
www.wvbop.com/

Wisconsin State Board of Pharmacy
Bureau Director
1400 E Washington
PO Box 8935
Madison, WI 53708-8935
Phone: 608/266-2112
Fax: 608/267-0644
www.drl.state.wi.us/

Wyoming State Board of Pharmacy
632 S David St
Casper, WY 82601
Phone: 307/234-0294
Fax: 307/234-7226
www.pharmacyboard.state.wy.us/

Chapter 7

Privacy of Patient Health Information

Chapter Outline

Learning Objectives

1. Identify the federal law established for maintaining privacy of patients' health information.
2. List the different entities handling patient health information that are covered by HIPAA.
3. Explain "protected health information."
4. Analyze examples of health information and determine if the information would or would not be covered by HIPAA.
5. Describe uses and disclosures of patient health information that are permitted by HIPAA.
6. Explain what to do when state and federal laws protecting the privacy of patient health information vary.
7. Compare and contrast day-to-day activities of a pharmacy technician that are covered by HIPAA with those that are not covered by HIPAA.

Introduction

Patients have a right of privacy for confidential health information, including the right to privacy and security of their personally identifiable health information maintained by pharmacies. Pharmacy technicians will have access to patients' private health information in most of their responsibilities such as dispensing prescriptions, contacting prescribers for refill authorizations, accepting prescriptions from patients, and delivering filled prescriptions to patients for pick-up. Accompanying the access to patient health information is the duty to maintain the required confidentiality and privacy of this information in accordance with state and federal laws and ethical responsibilities.

The private health information of patients is an obvious and necessary part of providing pharmacy patient care services and dispensing prescriptions. Pharmacy services could not be provided without necessary access and use of the patient's health information. It is part of virtually every aspect of pharmacy practice. By assisting pharmacists, pharmacy technicians will need to access and use a patient's private health information whether they are assisting with dispensing prescriptions, receiving prescriptions from patients, or contacting prescribers for refill authorizations. Privacy laws do not prohibit the necessary and customary use, disclosure, and communication of the patient's private health information because they are an essential part of providing patient care services. However, the privacy laws *do* require that health care providers, including pharmacies, comply with privacy and confidentiality laws and use reasonable safeguards to protect private patient health information.

Pharmacy records such as patient profiles and patient histories contain private patient health information used to provide pharmacy patient care services. Prescriptions that pharmacies receive, whether in writing, orally, or electronically, contain patients' private health information. Pharmacy computer systems record and maintain private patient prescription information and other private patient health information (e.g., laboratory results such as blood pressure or blood sugar results) or health information provided by patients (e.g., other diseases or conditions). Patient prescription container labels contain private health information by identifying the patient and his or her medication. Patient drug information materials handed out with dispensed prescriptions contain protected health information such as the patient name and prescribed medication. Patient billing records contain private health information. In short, virtually every record or document that pharmacies maintain and use will likely contain private health information for which privacy and confidentiality must be maintained. In common terms, this means that pharmacy technicians, pharmacists, pharmacy staff, and other health care providers need to be vigilant to maintain the privacy and confidentiality of the patient health information. This vigilance includes keeping pharmacy patient records secure in the pharmacy (such as ensuring that computers are locked and training employees in security procedures), not discarding patient information into regular trash receptacles, and keeping pharmacy conversations about patients from being overheard.

Patient private health information is part of most oral communications that occur in pharmacies and other health care settings where patient drug therapy and treatment are discussed. Oral communications in pharmacies also require steps to safeguard the privacy and confidentiality of patient health information. Examples of oral communications occurring in pharmacies include contacting the patient's physician by telephone to discuss the patient's drug therapy, counseling patients at the pharmacy counter about their prescription drug therapy, and telephoning physician offices for new prescriptions or prescription refill authorizations. Care must taken when engaging in these conversations to protect patient privacy and confidentiality.

Both state and federal laws establish requirements for maintaining privacy of patient health information. These laws apply to pharmacies as well as physicians and other health care providers. Health care providers, including pharmacists, pharmacy staff, and pharmacy technicians, are permitted to use and disclose patient health information as necessary to provide patient health care services. For example, a pharmacist is permitted to access, use, and disclose patient prescription information to dispense prescriptions, consult with health care providers on the patient's drug therapy, bill health care insurers to obtain payment for dispensed prescriptions, and for other necessary pharmacy patient care services and health care operations. The health information privacy laws also give patients specific rights regarding their health information, such as the right to obtain copies of their health records and to make corrections to their records.

 # Key Point

Health care providers, including pharmacists and pharmacy technicians, are permitted to access, use, and disclose patient health information as necessary to provide patient health care services.

It is important that pharmacy technicians, pharmacists, pharmacies, and other health care providers maintain the privacy and confidentiality of patients' medical information and health records as required by federal and state laws. The failure to comply with these laws may subject violators to significant penalties.

The primary federal law establishing health information privacy is the Health Insurance Portability and Accountability Act (HIPAA). States also have laws protecting the privacy and confidentiality of patient health and medical information. HIPAA sets the minimum requirements for privacy of patient personally identifiable health information. States may have greater protections for patient health information that must be followed. A discussion of all of the state privacy and confidentiality laws and their interaction with HIPAA is beyond the scope of this chapter. However, this chapter will discuss the important concepts in HIPAA for pharmacy technicians to know—that HIPAA sets the minimum protections and that state laws may provide greater protections than HIPAA.

 Key Point

The failure to comply with these laws may subject violators to signifi-cant penalties.

Federal Protections for Patient Health Information

The major federal law for privacy of health information, the Health Insurance Portability and Accountability Act ("HIPAA"), became effective in 2003 through final regulations. HIPAA set national standards for the privacy of patients' person-ally identifiable health information. HIPAA is a complicated law that covers the privacy and security of patient health information. This chapter focuses on the HIPAA privacy requirements. A review of the following key areas of HIPAA will assist pharmacy technicians in understanding the law:

▶ Health care providers and entities covered by HIPAA.
▶ Health information protected by HIPAA.
▶ Uses and disclosures of protected health information permitted under HIPAA.

"Who Is Covered by HIPAA?"

This federal law applies to health care providers, health plans, health care clear-inghouses such as billing services, and other entities that handle patient health information. Every health care provider is covered by HIPAA, including physi-cians, pharmacies, hospitals, clinics, and nursing homes and any other health care provider. The law applies to health plans that provide or pay for health care, such as health insurance companies, employer health plans, and federal and state programs that pay for health care (Medicare and Medicaid). HIPAA also covers entities that provide services for health care providers such as billing services for prescriptions, physicians, and other health care services. In addition, other busi-nesses that assist health care providers with processing health care information are covered by HIPAA (**Box 7-1**).

Box 7-1
Who Is Covered by HIPAA?

- Health plans that pay for health care products and services, including prescriptions
- Health care providers, including pharmacies
- Entities that provide services (e.g., billing)
- Other business associates that use or disclose health information in providing entities with whom the health care providers share the protected health information

---

 # Key Point

The HIPAA law applies to health care providers, health plans, health care clearinghouses such as billing services, and other entities that handle patient health information.

"What Patient Health Information Is Protected by HIPAA?"

The federal law protects *"individually identifiable health information"* whether it is oral, paper (e.g., a prescription or medical record), or electronic (e.g., in a pharmacy computer system or a hospital medical record system). Under HIPAA, the protected "individually identifiable health information" is called *"protected health information,"* which is commonly abbreviated as "PHI." Protected health information is any health information that includes patient identification information such as the patient's name, address, birth date, social security number, or data that could reasonably be used to identify the person and the patient's individual identifiable health information. Individually identifiable health information includes the person's past, present, or future physical or mental health or condition; the provision of health care to the persons; or the past, present, or future payment for the health care. It also includes information that identifies the person or could be used to identify the person. Examples of protected health information include pharmacy prescription records, including records in the pharmacy computer system, written prescriptions, and any records that the pharmacy keeps that contain PHI. It includes medical records (paper or electronic) kept by physician offices, hospitals, health clinics, and other health care entities. Billing records are considered protected health information. Oral communications may also contain protected health information such as conversations about a patient's health care and treatment or prescription drug therapy. For example, a pharmacist and a pharmacy technician may discuss a particular patient and the patient's prescription, or a pharmacist or pharmacy technician may call a physician's office about a patient's prescription.

Patient health information that does not personally identify the patient is not covered by the law. De-identified health information that does not identify the patient or provide a basis to identify the patient is not protected health information covered by HIPAA. For example, pharmacists and pharmacy technicians may discuss a particular drug therapy in general without mentioning a particular patient or any information that would enable the patient to be identified. General conversations of such a nature are not covered by HIPAA because they would not include any patient identifiable information even if they were overheard by another person. Nonetheless, when working in a pharmacy, it is always important to keep your conversations private and quiet even when specific patients are not mentioned due to the sensitivity of health matters. Another example is general patient educational leaflets that provide patients with information on how to use their medications but do not identify the patient or contain any patient identifiable information. They are not covered by HIPAA.

 Key Point

Patient health information that does not personally identify the patient or contain patient health information is not covered by HIPAA.

"What Are the Permitted Uses and Disclosures of Patient Health Information That Are Allowed by HIPAA?"

As mentioned above, the use and disclosure of patient identifiable information is necessary for providing pharmacy services and pharmacy operations. The basic concept of HIPAA is to protect patient health information while allowing permitted uses and disclosure of patient-protected health information for patient care, treatment, and health care operations (**Box 7-2**). Permitted uses and disclosures of patient health information are important because such information is necessary and essential for providing pharmacy services and other health care services. As a result, HIPAA permits the use and disclosure of patient-protected health information for a number of purposes such as patient treatment, payment for prescriptions, and health care operations (e.g., managing patient care) necessary for providing pharmacy services (**Box 7-3**).

Box 7-2
What Patient Health Information Is Covered by HIPAA?

- All patient information that a "covered entity" receives or creates that contains patient identifiable information
  - ◆ Patient information/data sheet filled out the first time a person visits a pharmacy
- Paper or electronic records that contain patient identifiable information
  - ◆ Prescriptions
  - ◆ Medical records
  - ◆ Patient profile on a computer system
- Oral communications that include patient identity information
  - ◆ Patient counseling
  - ◆ Prescription refill authorizations
  - ◆ New prescriptions being phoned in from the physician's office to the pharmacy
  - ◆ Phone call between a pharmacist and physician/nurse discussing a patient's treatment plan

---

 # Key Point

The basic concept of HIPAA is to protect patient personally identifiable health information while allowing permitted uses and disclosure of patient-protected health information for patient care, treatment, payment, and health care operations.

Pharmacies need to use and disclose patient health information for a number of pharmacy services, including dispensing prescriptions, billing the patient's insurance provider for payment, providing medication therapy management, and for other pharmacy patient services and health care operations. For example, permitted uses and disclosures allow pharmacies to check with insurance companies regarding drug coverage for a patient's prescription as well as contacting

---

Box 7-3
What Permitted Uses and Disclosures of Patient Health Information Are Allowed by HIPAA?

- To the person
- Patient treatment
- Payment (e.g., billing)
- Health care operations
- Other purposes such as research or public health

the patient's physician and other health care providers to discuss drug therapy, laboratory test results, and possible modification of the drug therapy.

HIPAA allows pharmacies and other health care providers to use professional judgment to decide when a disclosure is appropriate. For instance, HIPAA permits pharmacies to use the common practice of allowing a family member to pick up a prescription for the patient (e.g., a husband picking up a prescription for his wife). Pharmacy employers may have their own policies on persons authorized to pick up prescriptions. Pharmacy technicians should check with their pharmacy employer or the supervising pharmacist for any additional policies on persons that may pick up prescriptions for other persons.

In addition to the three questions discussed above, HIPAA includes other requirements for pharmacies and other health care providers. For instance, pharmacies, along with other health care providers, must notify their patients of their privacy rights (called "Notice of Privacy Practices") and obtain the signature of the patient's or the patient's authorized representative. Many pharmacies, physicians, and other health care providers supply written notice of privacy rights. Pharmacy technicians may have already seen the privacy notices that are provided by physicians' offices or hospitals, and been asked to sign them. As a pharmacy technician, you may be asked to provide a patient with a privacy notice and obtain the person's signature.

Additional HIPAA requirements exist. Pharmacy employees as well as other health care providers must receive training on the HIPAA privacy requirements. Each health care provider must have a *privacy officer* who is responsible for ensuring compliance with the required privacy practices. As a pharmacy technician, your pharmacy will have a privacy officer and provide you with privacy training and information on its privacy practices.

Pharmacy technicians have an important role in protecting the privacy of patient health information in the pharmacy. Paying close attention to how you handle patient health information and following your pharmacy's policies and procedures on patient privacy are important steps to complying with federal and state laws and being continually aware of respecting patient privacy.

State Laws Protecting Patient Health Information

States also have laws protecting the privacy of patient health information. The state laws vary considerably. It is beyond the scope of this chapter to discuss and compare the state patient privacy laws due to their complexities. Nevertheless, some basic considerations are important for pharmacy technicians to understand. The federal HIPAA law sets the *minimum* protections for patient health information and pharmacies, and other covered health care providers and entities must comply with HIPAA. If state laws provide less protection than HIPAA, the federal HIPAA protections would apply. However, the reverse is true where the state law provides greater protections for patient health information. If the state patient privacy law is stronger than HIPAA, then the stronger state law protections would apply along with the HIPAA requirements. Although this is a complicated area of law, the significant points for pharmacy technicians to be aware of are that 1) patient health information is covered by privacy protections and that 2) it is important to always take steps to safeguard the security and privacy of patients' health information.

 Key Point

The federal HIPAA law sets the *minimum* protections for patient health information and pharmacies, and other covered health care providers and entities must comply with HIPAA.

Summary

As a pharmacy technician, you have an important role in maintaining patient privacy protections. Day-to-day steps that pharmacy technicians take to protect patient health information are essential such as properly disposing of materials that contain identifiable patient health information, maintaining appropriate privacy of communications about patients, maintaining security of pharmacy computer systems (e.g., not sharing your password and locking computers as necessary), and maintaining respect for patient privacy by not discussing patient information with others outside the pharmacy or where it may be overheard.

Federal and state laws establish privacy and confidentiality protections for patient health information, including prescription and health information maintained by pharmacies. Pharmacists, pharmacy technicians, and other pharmacy personnel have legal and ethical responsibilities to maintain confidentiality and privacy of patients' protected health information. The major federal act for privacy of health information is the Health Insurance Portability and Accountability Act ("HIPAA"). States also have laws protecting the privacy of patient health information. HIPAA, the federal law, sets the minimum confidentiality protections for protected health information. Some state laws may provide greater privacy protections than HIPAA. Pharmacy records contain private health information, including prescriptions, patient profiles and histories, the patient's prescription containers, written information provided by pharmacies, and other material that identifies the patient and his or her medication. Private patient health information may also be part of oral or telephone conversations that discuss a particular patient. Pharmacy staff, including pharmacy technicians, should use continual care to maintain and safeguard the security and privacy of patient-protected health information in compliance with federal and state patient confidentiality and privacy laws.

Self-Assessment Questions

1. What is HIPPA and what does it do?
2. What is PHI?
3. What oral communications are covered by HIPAA?
4. If the state privacy law is stronger and more stringent than HIPAA, which law is applied?
5. Do pharmacy technicians have as much responsibility to protect the privacy of patients as pharmacists?

Self-Assessment Answers

Chapter 1

1. Sources of oversight and standards include federal laws and regulations, state laws and regulations, professional practice standards, ethical principles, case law
2. Drug Enforcement Administration (DEA)
3. The federal Omnibus Budget Reconciliation Act of 1990 (commonly called "OBRA '90") was the first federal law to address the standards of practice for pharmacists.
4. In the late 1970s, two national pharmacy organizations, the American Pharmacists Association (APhA) and the American Association of Colleges of Pharmacy (AACP), worked together to create the APhA/AACP Standards of Practice of the Profession of Pharmacy. The national professional association for health-system pharmacists, the American Society of Health-System Pharmacists (ASHP), also developed professional standards for pharmacists.
5. The state Board of Pharmacy

Chapter 2

1. Legislatures make laws or statutes by introducing and passing legislation.
2. State governments are comprised of the same three branches as the federal government: legislative, executive, and judicial.
3. Federal legislation can be introduced by a member of Congress: a Senator or a Representative.
4. These are examples of federal administrative or regulatory agencies.
5. Pharmacy practice laws and regulations

Chapter 3

1. The FDCA includes comprehensive requirements for drug manufacturing, distribution, labeling, and marketing in the United States.
2. The package insert is intended for pharmacists, physicians, and health care providers.
3. Also known as the Prescription Drug Amendment, the Durham–Humphrey Amendment requires that certain drugs be dispensed only pursuant to a prescription and required that any refills be authorized either in the original prescription or by the prescriber.
4. The FDA enforces the FDCA.
5. MTM stands for Medication Therapy Management and is a service provided to patients by either pharmacists or other health care providers who review a patient's prescription drug therapy.

Chapter 4

1. The FDA ensures the safety and efficacy of human drugs made and distributed in the United States through its drug approval process.
2. After a drug company's drug patent expires, it is legal for other drug companies to manufacture the same drug using the identical active ingredient as the brand name drug. These are known as generically equivalent drugs. Before a generic drug manufacturer is permitted to market and distribute a generically equivalent drug, the drug manufacturer must establish to FDA that its generic drug is therapeutically equivalent to the brand name drug.
3. The generic substitution laws and regulations allow pharmacists to substitute therapeutically equivalent generic drugs for prescribed brand name drugs unless the prescriber requests the brand name drug.
4. OTC labeling is designed for the patient or consumer.
5. Drug expiration dates are derived from drug stability studies.

Chapter 5

1. Controlled substances require more stringent controls by federal and state laws because of the potential for misuse, abuse, diversion, and addiction.
2. The CSA is the Controlled Substances Act, and it establishes comprehensive controls over the manufacture, import, export, distribution, ordering, dispensing, and prescribing of controlled substances.
3. A pharmacy, pharmacist, or physician must be registered with the DEA to have access to controlled substances.

4. Federal law requires that if a controlled substance is stolen or lost from a pharmacy, the pharmacy must immediately report the theft or loss to the DEA using DEA form 106 "Report of Theft or Loss of Controlled Substances." State laws may also have requirements for pharmacy reporting and other responsibilities in the event of lost or stolen controlled substances.
5. The federal CMEA is the Combat Methamphetamine Epidemic Act, and it limits sales of products containing pseudoephedrine, ephedrine, and phenylpropanolamine to 3.6 grams daily due to concerns that these products were being used to illegally manufacture methamphetamine.

Chapter 6

1. The state Board of Pharmacy has the authority, oversight, and enforcement power over the licensure and registration of pharmacy technicians with the state.
2. Other possible state requirements for pharmacy technicians include: high school graduate or equivalent; a minimum age requirement; good moral character; no conviction of a drug-related felony; specific education and training; examinations, certification, criminal background checks; continuing education.
3. Pharmacy technician ratios comprise the number of pharmacy technicians allowed to assist a pharmacist in the pharmacy.
4. In general, pharmacy technicians are not permitted to perform tasks that require the professional judgment, education, and training of a pharmacist. State pharmacy laws may place other restrictions on the tasks that pharmacy technicians are permitted to perform or not perform.
5. The Pharmacy Technician Certification Board.

Chapter 7

1. HIPAA is the federal Health Insurance Portability and Accountability Act and is the primary federal law that establishes privacy protections for patient health information.
2. PHI stands for "protected health information." PHI is any health information that includes patient identification information such as the patient identification numbers, patient name, address, birth date, and social security number; or information that could be reasonably used to identify the patient.
3. HIPPA covers oral communications that include patient identity information such as conversations between the patient and pharmacist during patient counseling, prescription refill authorizations, and new prescriptions being

phoned in from the physician's office to the pharmacy where the identity of the patient and the patient health information may be overheard. Other examples are telephone conversations between a pharmacist and physician or nurse where the patient's identity and treatment plan are discussed.

4. The federal HIPAA law sets the minimum protections for patient health information. If the state law is more stringent, it takes precedence over HIPPA and the stronger state law protections would apply.

5. Yes, pharmacy technicians must adhere to HIPPA and all other patient privacy laws, both state and federal.

Index